D1111786

STRATEGIC
RESEARCH

STRATEGIC RESEARCH

A Practical Handbook for Phase IIIB and Phase IV Clinical Studies

HUGO STEPHENSON, MD

QUINTILES TRANSNATIONAL CORPORATION
RESEARCH TRIANGLE PARK, NORTH CAROLINA

Published 2005 by Quintiles Transnational
4709 Creekstone Drive
Durham, North Carolina 27703

ISBN 0-9770317-0-5

This book has been composed in Minion.

Printed in the United States of America

1 3 5 7 9 10 8 6 4 2

Contents

Part III: Unique Study Dynamics

Part IV: Special Cases of Strategic Research

• • • • •

STRATEGIC
RESEARCH

Acknowledgments

I WOULD LIKE TO THANK the following people for contributing their time and knowledge to the process of creating this book on Phase IIIB and IV studies. From Quintiles: Karen Brown, Director, Corporate Marketing; Elisa Cascade, Vice President of Corporate Development; Lorne Cheeseman, Head of Quality Assurance; Oren Cohen, MD, Chief Medical and Scientific Officer; Dick Jones, Senior Director, Corporate Communication; Lauren Kim, Associate, SRS Analytical Services; Elizabeth Lapetina, Project Specialist, SRS Analytical Services; Hervé Laurent, Senior Vice President, SRS Europe; Dana Marohn, Research Analyst, SRS Analytical Services; Axel Olsen, PhD, Executive Director, Data Analytics and Consulting; Ilina Sen, Research Analyst, SRS Analytical Services; John Russell, Executive Vice-President, General Counsel & Chief Administrative Officer; and Nancy Strehlow, Special Counsel for Health Law and Policy.

I would also like to thank the writing and production team. For writing and project management, Alexi Assmus, PhD, Assmus Group, LLC; for interior illustrations, Dimitri Karetnikov; for front cover design concept, Jim Phillips, Chief Creative Guy, Bailey+Phillips Group; for cover and interior design, Sarah Stengle; and for copyediting, Tim Sullivan.

I would specifically like to thank Karen Brown, Oren Cohen, and Nancy Strehlow who have patiently provided input and feedback throughout the drafting process, often at very short notice.

I would also like to thank Professor John McNeil, who introduced me as a medical student to the entrepreneurial possibilities associated with strategic research, and Dr. Dennis Gillings, whose vision for global pharmaceutical outsourcing has allowed me to consolidate best practices in strategic research from around the world.

Most importantly I would like to thank my wife, Melanie, and our children and parents, who have not only accepted my prolonged absences required to write this book but have supported me in my long—and sometimes demanding—transition from medical practice to applied clinical research.

Foreword

SINCE THE LATE 1990s, the pharmaceutical industry has recognized the increasing importance of trials conducted after the submission of a marketing authorization. While spending in Phases II and III has grown about 7 percent each year, spending on postmarketing clinical research is growing at an annual rate of 20 percent.* Our industry has learned—both through good fortune and expensive mistakes—that the conduct of peri- and post-marketing studies requires a special approach and a new set of skills and tools different than those required for drug approval. Most importantly, we have learned that this research brings with it a new set of risks.

Part I of the book introduces the concept of Phase IIIB and IV research, also know as strategic research, and can be read by a general audience. Parts II–IV form a practical handbook to this type of research and will be valuable to project managers and research associates embarking on these studies. Part II addresses how companies can design strategic research programs to optimally advance and defend a product's position with scientific integrity; we also reflect upon safety, risk management, and regulatory issues. Part III explores the practical application and mechanics of these studies, and Part IV treats special cases of strategic research. The appendix explains how the Anti-kickback Statute and the False Claims Act apply to strategic research in the United States.

*Center Watch, Inc. Presentation at CBI's 3rd Annual Phase IV Clinical Trials Conference (tracked over the period 1999 to 2001); September 23, 2002.

The book addresses several audiences: those with existing clinical trials experience who wish to understand more about the special nature of Phase IIIB and IV research—what makes it different, and how these differences can impact study design and conduct; members of the brand team charged with designing research plans; and corporate leaders who want to maximize the effectiveness of their research investments.

Since accidentally migrating from medical practice to clinical research in the 1990s, I have been fascinated by science that grabs the public interest—science that changes prescribing and patient-care patterns, monitors public safety, and drives measurable community health improvement.

I hope that in reading this book you will come to appreciate the opportunities offered by strategic research. My broader goal is to foster an understanding of the field that will help ensure that patients, payors, and physicians have the information they require to make good treatment decisions.

HUGO STEPHENSON, MD

I   Introduction

1   What Is Strategic Research?

CLINICAL TRIALS ARE the scientifically rigorous way to measure whether new drugs are safe and effective in patients. Since the first randomized controlled trial (RCT) conducted in 1948, regulatory agencies have used clinical trials to determine whether a new drug is ready for the public.[1] Over the past decade, however, it has become clear that the clinical trials required by regulatory agencies for approval leave many important questions unanswered. The pharmaceutical industry now regularly conducts clinical research after the submission of a new drug application to provide information to providers, patients, and payors about drugs that are close to receiving marketing approval or that the general public is already using.

These studies are called Phase IIIB and IV studies because they follow the Phase I–III clinical trials required by regulatory agencies for initial registration. Increasingly known as *strategic research* they have become a critical part of every peri- and post-marketing product strategy. Companies choose to conduct them for many reasons, such as monitoring product safety and discovering new uses for the drug once it is on the market. These studies address a larger audience than the earlier phase studies, including doctors, patients, insurers, and the media, in addition to the regulatory agencies, and take a wider variety of forms because they are not restricted to the randomized controlled format that regulators require for drug approval.

In the past, this research has been negatively associated with "seeding" studies whose main goal was to give physicians an incentive to start prescribing a drug. Companies would design such "studies" to gather trivial data that resulted in scripts for thousands and thousands of new patients. Since the passage of the Medicare and Medicaid Protection Act of 1987, the regulatory environment in the United States has become hostile to these types of seeding studies, and reputable organizations no longer conduct them. Similar trends are emerging in Europe. With the decline of seeding studies and greater emphasis on product safety has come greater recognition of the scientific importance of strategic research.

Scientifically rigorous Phase IIIB and IV studies have had significant impact on the marketplace. In the late 1990s, Warner-Lambert and Pfizer used such studies to show that Lipitor, a new cholesterol-lowering drug, led to improved health outcomes as opposed to other drugs already on the market. Lipitor became a new blockbuster drug, while its competitors, Pravachol and Zocor, suffered declining sales. In contrast, Merck's analysis of data from its APPROVe study resulted in the withdrawal of the blockbuster drug Vioxx. This Phase IIIB trial for a new indication famously confirmed cardiovascular risks of long-term exposure. As these examples show, strategic studies can make or break a product.

Two Stages of Drug Development: Registration and Strategic Research

Today's regulatory environment has divided the drug development process into two stages: obtaining approval to sell a product, followed by generating the information providers and patients need to use the drug most effectively.

The first stage of the drug development process—which includes preclinical research, and Phase I, Phase II, and Phase III trials—focuses on obtaining product approval. Following testing on animals, the early phase trials begin by investigating human pharmacology to determine toxicity (Phase I), explore effectiveness and identify an appropriate dose regime (Phase II), and confirm effectiveness in large populations (Phase III).[2] Often referred to as *registration research*, these studies generate data for submission in support of an new drug application and are pivotal to any product approval decision.

Since registration research primarily targets the information needs of regulators, it is generally constrained by guidelines, advisories, and past agency decisions that limit research to tightly designed clinical trials. Pharmaceutical companies invest in this clinical research to meet regulatory requirements for drug approval but find that these studies are often too limited in duration of treatment or diversity of patient population to effectively evaluate safety in the general population. Even after research findings satisfy regulatory agencies, many questions remain unanswered. It is here that Phase IIIB and IV studies play a large role.

With the Food and Drug Administration's Acting Commissioner Lester M. Crawford acknowledging a 50 percent product attrition rate during Phase III alone,[3] most companies are reluctant to expand the focus of their research investment until they are confident that a regulatory agency will approve their product. Companies wait for a thumbs-up from regulatory agencies before investing in a second stage of research.

Once a manufacturer no longer needs to focus solely on product approval, they can turn to addressing unanswered questions that could impact optimal use of a product through Phase IIIB and IV programs. This second stage of research has been collectively referred to as late phase, late stage, or peri- and post-marketing, but since market forces can affect the mechanics of this research and the results of these studies can influence market behavior, the industry has come to call it *strategic research*.*

Phase IIIB and IV studies cover a spectrum of designs, and range from highly controlled, randomized studies, identical in type to registration studies, to retrospective studies using preexisting databases that can be completed in less than three months. Patient numbers can range from 200 to 100,000, often targeting diverse patient groups including children, the elderly, and patients with complex comorbidities.

Six to eighteen months before anticipated launch, many companies begin reviewing their data from registration trials in a market context. In developing a brand strategy, a company must judge whether their early-phase research provides the public with enough information to ensure that their drug is most effectively used. Companies can *strategically* use Phase IIIB and IV research to fill critical information gaps before and immediately after launch.

All gaps are not necessarily closed before launch, and new gaps will emerge during the drug's lifetime. Pharmaceutical companies must regularly review what additional information patients, physicians, insurers, and the media require, making Phase IIIB and IV research an ongoing concern.

Questions answered by Phase IIIB and IV research include: What can patients and physicians expect from using a product? Does this vary from patient to patient? How does it compare with its competitors? What is the drug's safety profile in large populations and over long periods of use? How cost effective is treatment, and what pricing strategy is likely to result in most effective market uptake? Could the product be used to treat other conditions? Could restriction of the product's label limit potential medico-legal liability?

*As an example of how market forces can affect the mechanics of the study: if a product becomes reimbursed during the course of a study, it suddenly becomes much harder to recruit patients.

Phase IIIB

The moment the manufacturer applies for marketing authorization for a particular product, all ongoing clinical research not conducted in line with an approved product label becomes, in industry parlance, Phase IIIB research.* Pre-approval Phase IIIB studies occur while the regulatory agency is reviewing the submission and usually focus on generating additional data to support the product's anticipated launch. Such activities include observational studies that inform treatment guidelines or randomized controlled studies that compare the efficacy of a product against its market competitors. These activities can also include expanded access programs that offer products before they are approved to severely ill patients.

CHALLENGING MARKET BEHAVIOR

Preparing for product launches across Europe throughout the year, AstraZeneca announced data from the 2,431-patient STELLAR study in April 2003.[4] By demonstrating that Crestor had greater dose-for-dose efficacy in reducing cholesterol than any of its major competitors, the results of this randomized controlled trial created an opportunity for AstraZeneca to challenge the normal prescribing pattern of physicians.[5]

Post-approval Phase IIIB studies investigate the use of approved drugs outside the terms of their approved product label. They are usually conducted to explore new therapeutic opportunities or support changes to the product label. Geodon, a commonly used anti-psychotic drug, was introduced to the market for the treatment of schizophrenia in February 2001. As a result of Phase IIIB research investigating new indications, Geodon received approval for treatment of bipolar mania in August 2004.

---

* While Phase IIIB is not a definition formally used by regulatory authorities, the industry does use the term to describe additional therapeutic exploratory and confirmatory studies conducted after the primary regulatory dossier has been submitted.

Phase IIIB studies, both pre- and post-approval, use products in ways that have not been approved and are therefore associated with greater potential patient risk than studies performed on approved drugs for already approved uses, called Phase IV research. As a result, Phase IIIB studies usually involve checks and balances to ensure patient safety, including tighter enrollment criteria for subject participation, more frequent and detailed patient follow-up, more detailed adverse event tracking, and more frequent monitoring activities than are normally required in Phase IV.

Phase IV

Phase IV research investigates approved products used in line with their approval labels. Examples include randomized, controlled trials that are conducted to address questions about comparative efficacy, tolerability, and cost effectiveness of different treatment approaches. Because physicians are prescribing these approved drugs under uncontrolled conditions, observational studies that capture naturalistic data about treatment outcomes over time can also be performed, informing treatment guidelines and best practices. Many post-marketing safety studies take this form. If a drug has been available for a significant period of time, data may be available retrospectively from patient records and files. Note that Phase IIIB and IV trials often occur in parallel, as companies seek to explore expanded uses of the drug at the same time as solidifying the scientific basis for their product's existing claims.

· · · · ·

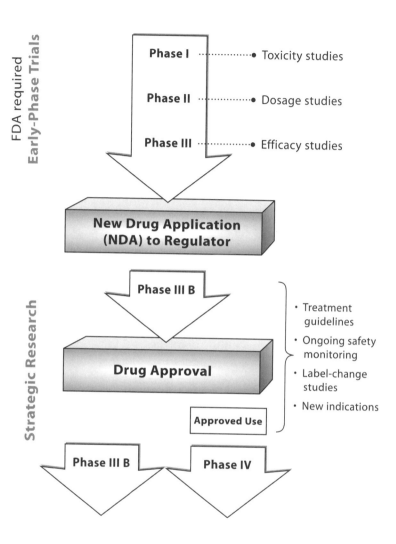

FIGURE 1.1. PHASES OF CLINICAL RESEARCH
Phases IIIB and IV studies, those conducted after the filing of a new drug application, are increasingly being described as strategic research given their role in supporting product strategy.

IDENTIFYING FAVORABLE PRODUCT CHARACTERISTICS

Although numerous drugs are available for the treatment of schizophrenia, each product has different strengths and weaknesses that psychiatrists must balance when selecting the right treatment for each patient. The more information available, the more effectively patients can be matched with the most appropriate treatment. In December 2004, Eli Lilly & Co. published data from a large three-year naturalistic Phase IV study, SCAP (Schizophrenia Care and Assessment Program), suggesting that patients receiving long-term treatment with Lilly's antipsychotic Zyprexa were at lower risk of exhibiting violent behavior than those receiving Janssen's Risperdal.[6] Findings like these can be very powerful in supporting a physician's choice of anti-psychotic treatment.

Companies frequently conduct Phase IV studies to monitor product safety under real-world conditions. These studies can avoid the selection bias associated with registration research by involving large numbers of patients who have complicating factors that would have barred them from participating in the controlled Phase II or III trials. Only when a product is used outside the tightly controlled clinical trial conditions of earlier registration research does its true benefits and hidden dangers become apparent. Phase IV trials can also play a part in a company's appropriate due diligence to ensure that medicines are used most effectively and safely within the community, minimizing harm to patients and ultimately medico-legal risk.

• • • • •

SAFETY LIMITATIONS OF REGISTRATION RESEARCH
A prime example of how registration trials can miss significant safety issues is the case of Rezulin, a diabetes drug that began to be used widely after its introduction in early 1997. Unfortunately, the number of patients treated in registration studies was insufficient to effectively quantify the product's risk of severe liver damage. These controlled clinical trials only reported rare cases of reversible jaundice by the time that the product was approved in March 1997. But by October 1997, after less than six months of real world use, 35 cases of idiosyncratic hepatocellular injury (resulting in one transplant and one death) had been reported to the FDA. Rezulin was withdrawn from the market in 2000 after an FDA review of safety data showed it to be more toxic to the liver than the newer drugs in the same class, Avandia and Actos.[7]

Conclusion

In the past, some late-phase clinical studies gave the field a bad name because they were conducted with the express purpose of getting physicians to prescribe new drugs. As these seeding studies have become illegal in today's more stringent regulatory environment, scientifically valid Phase IIIB and IV studies, always important, have begun to receive more attention. They are used to provide information on safety issues, to assist in the development of more extensive treatment guidelines, to explore new indications, and to compare drugs within the same class with an eye to what patients and payors feel is important about a drug's effects and costs.

Strategic research allows manufacturers to address questions about their products that remain unanswered at the time of registration, and that may arise later in a product's lifecycle. As the industry continues to face greater scrutiny, sponsors are discovering that providing more scientific information to a discerning public, to health care organizations and to regulatory agencies is a good investment.

References

1. Hill AB. The clinical trial. N Engl J Med. 1952;247:113–19.

2. International Conference on Harmonisation of Technical Requirements for Registration of Pharmaceuticals for Human Use. ICH Harmonised Tripartite Guideline: General Considerations for Clinical Trials (E8). Recommended for Adoption at Step 4 of the ICH Process on July 17, 1997 by the ICH Steering Committee, pp. 6–7.

3. Presentation by Lester M. Crawford, for Bank of America Securities Health Care Institutional Investor Conference, July 7, 2004. www.fda.gov/oc/speeches/2004/bascrty0707.html.*

4. AstraZeneca Press Release, New Crestor Data at ACC Meeting Confirm Superior Product Profile, April 2, 2003.

5. Jones PH, Davidson MH, Stein EA, Bays HE, McKenney JM, Miller E, Cain VA, Blasetto JW; STELLAR Study Group. Comparison of the efficacy and safety of rosuvastatin versus atorvastatin, simvastatin, and pravastatin across doses (STELLAR Trial). Am J Cardiol 2003 Jul 15;92(2):152–60.

6. Swanson JW et al. Reducing violence risk in persons with schizophrenia: olanzapine versus risperidone. J Clin Psychiatry 2004 Dec;65(12):1666–73.

7. HHS News, FDA. Rezulin to be withdrawn from the market; March 21, 2000. Available at http://www.fda.gov/bbs/topics/NEWS/NEW00721.html.*

Note: All citations to websites listed in this book were verified in May of 2005.

2   Why Is It Growing?

UNTIL THE MID-1990s, the prescribing preferences of individual physicians collectively influenced the success or failure of new products. While individual physicians continue to be central to a drug's success, as demonstrated by the enduring number of field-based pharmaceutical sales representatives, they no longer represent decision-making units acting in isolation. Patients and patient advocacy groups, health insurance organizations, pharmacists, nurses and nurse practitioners, regulatory agencies, politicians, and even the media have become active stakeholders in the pharmaceutical market. The pharmaceutical industry's effort to address growing interest in their products is fueling a growth in Phase IV research funding of over 20 percent each year.[1] Estimates for Phase IIIB and IV spending in 2004 put it at $3.7 billion, and predictions are it will increase to over $5 billion by 2008.[2]

More Public Awareness

Patients have become increasingly sophisticated and pro-active in their own health care. Internet discussion groups, websites, and patient support groups have all created spaces for patients to come together and learn about their disease and its treatment. For the very committed, resources like Medline, widely available at public libraries, make it possible to follow the results of clinical studies. Direct-to-consumer advertising, which has been allowed on tele-

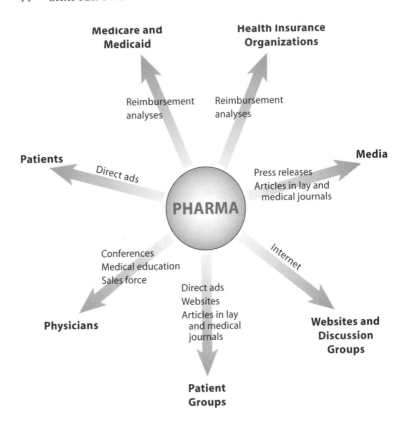

Figure 2. The large number of stakeholders today distinguishes the industry from the past when physicians and drug manufacturers were the primary players in the pharmaceutical industry. Strategic research is now used to address the different information needs of these groups.

vision and radio in the United States since the late nineties, has had an enormous and measurable influence on patients' desire for and access to certain drugs. Of patients who asked their doctor to prescribe a drug they had seen advertised, 44 percent received it.[3]

As an increasingly educated community has taken a greater interest in healthcare, the media has taken a leading role in providing relevant information. Health care issues have become big news. Prominent health writers like Jane Brody of the *New York Times* do their own extensive research into clinical trials and survey medical opinion on a new drug before recommending it to their readers.

A recent story illustrates the power of this trend. The release of results from the Women's Health Initiative (WHI) study in 2002, a Phase IV trial partially funded by Wyeth and conducted by the National Institutes of Health (NIH) to investigate long-term combination hormone replacement therapy (HRT) for the treatment of cardiovascular and fracture risk in postmenopausal women, generated a significant level of public discussion.[4] The trial uncovered an association between long-term combination HRT use and an increased risk of breast cancer, generating explosive publicity; in the months after publication of the results, hundreds of stories appeared in U.S. newspapers and magazines addressing the risks of therapy. The publicity surrounding the WHI study is credited with instantly wiping out more than $850 million from the global HRT market.[5]

Not surprisingly, a recently published study found that media reports on the WHI study had a significant influence on women's use of HRT.[6] More than 50 percent of women discontinued or curtailed HRT use after reading about the study results, even those using estrogen alone (for which no elevated risk was reported in the study), and those receiving short-term treatment for management of menopausal symptoms (which the study was not designed to investigate).

Today public perceptions of medical treatment can change so quickly and unpredictably that successful companies need to do more clinical research than in the past to remain ahead of the issues. Could additional research focused on short-term HRT have helped women feel more comfortable continuing their therapy? Could data linking termination of treatment for menopausal symptoms with increased incidence of depression, or decreased quality of life, have altered the decisions of women and their physicians?

In the past, physicians were the primary targets of scientific communications. Today, with an increasingly sophisticated public and active media, how pharmaceutical companies choose to address the evolving information needs of new stakeholders through Phase IIIB and IV research can dramatically influence the reception of their products.

Increased Focus on Drug Safety

The cost of lawsuits against the pharmaceutical industry has forced many companies to adopt focused risk management strategies at the highest levels. Wyeth's legal challenges relating to Fenfluramine and Dexfenfluramine (Fen-Phen) have demonstrated how quickly and high pharmaceutical settlements can add up. Costs to Wyeth are now over $20 billion in money either already paid out or set aside to settle ongoing lawsuits.[7]

Because drug approval represents a balance between protecting public safety and making new products available for patients to use, products are generally approved before their safety profile is fully characterized. Small patient numbers, constraints on patient diversity, and short-term use of therapy associated with Phase II and III studies limit the ability of registration research to detect serious side effects. These unknown side effects may occur in special populations, after prolonged periods of exposure, or with an incidence lower than 1 event per 1000 patients treated. Post-approval studies are therefore necessary to catch unexpected safety events that only emerge when the product is used in a large, diverse population for long periods of time.

LATENT SIDE EFFECTS

Some side effects reveal themselves only after long periods of exposure to a drug. Lung cancers appear years after patients first start smoking. Mesothelioma usually appears more than 20 years after exposure to asbestos dust. As a less well-known example, in 2004 researchers from Brigham and Women's Hospital in Boston published data from a prospective study of almost 1,700 women that demonstrated a strong association between frequent acetaminophen use and a 30 percent decline in renal function over an 11-year period. Most drugs in use today have not been available for twenty years, let alone been taken by the same patient for such a long period of time. How many long term side effects will reveal themselves only after decades of patient exposure?[8]

The case of spironolactone, a potassium-sparing diuretic, nicely illustrates how results from randomized studies cannot always be generalized beyond the controlled patient populations enrolled. The Randomized Aldactone Evaluation Study (RALES) demonstrated that treatment with spironolactone substantially reduced morbidity and mortality in a controlled population of patients with severe heart failure.[9] Not surprisingly, clinical guidelines were amended across the world to reflect this conclusion until, in mid 2004, a Canadian study showed that spironolactone had led to more deaths from dangerously high levels of potassium than would have been expected. With a higher incidence of age- and diabetes-related renal impairment than the study population, more patients in the real world were found to be developing dangerously high potassium levels. Those physicians who continue to use spironolcatone now monitor potassium levels much more aggressively.

Recognizing deficiencies in the registration research process, regulators are increasingly demanding post-marketing research as a condition of drug approval. More than 60 percent of FDA approvals in 2003 required at least one post-marketing research commitment as a condition of approval. The FDA register recorded more than 1,479 open post-marketing research commitments as of September 30, 2004.[10] As juries increasingly focus on studies that could have been done but were not, and public pressure on regulators to focus on drug safety continues to grow, we can only anticipate rapid expansion of Phase IIIB and IV research activities as an important foundation of corporate and public risk management.

Greater Pharmaceutical Competition

While the sequencing of the human genome raised widespread hope for a revolution in the prevention and treatment of disease, the beginning of the new millennium has marked a slowdown in novel drug and biologic submissions to regulatory agencies worldwide.[11] While our scientific knowledge has been increasing exponentially, the expanding gap between the laboratory and the bedside has been accompanied by products going off-patent at a faster rate than the industry's ability to replace them. Faced with escalating costs of drug development and pressure to replenish their patent-protected product portfolios, it has been a safer bet for companies to develop follow-up products to successful drugs than to pioneer truly novel treatments.

While regulators review critical pathways in search of obstacles whose elimination might kickstart a new wave of drug development, the industry faces the growing challenge of differentiating their products in a crowded market of generic alternatives and competing products that share similar approval labels. By generating data to support competitive product positioning through label changes, comparative effectiveness, cost/benefit analysis, and therapeutic guideline development, Phase IIIB and IV research is becoming increasingly important for companies that need to identify and defend product opportunities.

BIG OPPORTUNITIES, BIG INVESTMENT
Attempts to secure the now $30 billion lipid lowering market have stimulated some of the largest and most expensive Phase IIIB and IV trials in the history of the pharmaceutical industry including LIPID[12] (9,014 patients), MIRACL[13] (3,086), STEL-LAR[14] (2,268), CARE[15] (4,159), WOSCOPS[16] (6,595), 4S[17] (4,444), AFSCAPS/TexCAPS[18] (6605), HPS[19] (20,536), ASCOT[20] (10,305), CARDS[21] (2,838), ASAP[22] (325), JUPITER[23] (15,000), PROVE-IT[24] (4,162), REVERSAL[25] (654), and ALLIANCE[26] (2,442). These studies, involving more than 75,000 patients, have contributed significantly to our current treatment of high cholesterol and the management of cardiovascular risk, but at no small cost. With industry estimates suggesting a fully loaded cost per patient of between $3,000 and $5,000 in 1999, these trials alone reflect an industry investment in peri- and post-approval research of well over $300m.[27]

Increased Focus on Pharmaceutical Pricing

The pharmaceutical industry in the United States has been the beneficiary of generous policies toward drug pricing. In the world's largest pharmaceutical market, pricing strategy involves the balance of price against demand to establish an optimal price point. Even so, U.S. health insurance companies, preferred provider networks, and government agencies that are responsible for health costs at both the federal and state level have become ever more sensitive to drug prices. In the United States, the spiraling cost of drugs, particularly for seniors, has become a major political issue.

Other major markets, including Europe, Canada, Australia, and Japan, have adopted a centralized government formulary approach. In these markets, the single buyer is well positioned to negotiate. Pharmaceutical companies must justify a product's price by demonstrating its potential economic benefits (e.g., decreasing other healthcare costs or increasing work productivity). These market dynamics have created a significant cost differential between products sold in the United States and those sold overseas.

As pharmaceutical competition increases and the incremental benefit associated with new medications continues to diminish, formularies in the United States find themselves in a better position to negotiate prices than in the past. For instance, most formularies now demand generic substitution where available. And as competition increases within therapeutic classes, formularies can negotiate significant discounts when selecting a preferred product. Pharmaceutical subsidy for the aged through Medicare is already increasing collective formulary negotiating power, and the barriers to importation that protect U.S. pharmaceutical sales are under increasing pressure for reform.

In this new world, most pharmaceutical companies recognize a convergence between historic U.S. approaches to pharmaceutical pricing and the cost-benefit rationale successfully applied elsewhere. Cost-benefit-based price justification is already practiced in the United States, and price controls are inevitable at some point in the future.

• • • • •

INCREASING FOCUS ON HEALTH ECONOMICS

Merck's Phase IIIB Scandinavian Simvastatin Survival Study (4S) was the first to demonstrate that a statin could help save lives and prevent heart attacks in patients with high cholesterol and heart disease. Addressing a group of executives in November 2000, Merck's chairman, Raymond Gilmartin, responded to concerns about increasing pressure on drug companies to prove the value of their medicines by citing analyses of 4S data which demonstrated that ZOCOR treatment could lower hospitalization rates and reduce the need for costly cardiovascular procedures.[28]

As the spotlight on pricing grows, drug companies are focusing more energy on research to demonstrate that their products perform differently than inexpensive generics and less expensive competitors. As new treatments emerge for previously undertreated or non–life threatening conditions, companies will find it increasingly necessary to justify the cost of additional treatment against economic benefit.

Conclusion

With increasing patient participation in healthcare decision-making, it is becoming more important for pharmaceutical companies to address the gap between the information generated by registration studies and the needs of public and media stakeholders. Phase IIIB and IV research provides a ready tool for such an approach. Regulatory approval was once the final hurdle to product success; today it simply gets the company a seat at the table. Facing growing pressure to demonstrate value in a crowded market filled with generic competitors, and growing public concern regarding the safety of new medicines, the most effective companies will continue to conduct increasing amounts of strategic research to ensure that their products receive the greatest possible opportunities in a crowded and price sensitive market.

References

1. Center Watch, Inc. Presentation at CBI's 3rd Annual Phase IV Clinical Trials Conference (tracked over the period 1999 to 2001); September 23, 2002.

2. Jefferies & Company. Contract Research Industry Comprehensive Update: Can CROs Outperform Their Customers Again. Pharmacuetical Services Quarterly Preview January 19, 2005.

3. The Henry J. Kaiser Family Foundation. Understanding the Effects of Direct-to-Consumer Prescription Drug Advertising, November 2001, p. 3.

4. Rossouw JE, Anderson GL, Prentice RL et al. Risks and benefits of estrogen plus progestin in healthy postmenopausal women: principal results from the Women's Health Initiative randomized controlled trial. JAMA 2002;288:321–33.

5. Osteoporosis and HRT: Novel Osteoporosis Drugs Counter Generic Threat While HRT Players Regroup and Move Forward, Datamonitor, October 2004.

6. McIntosh J, Blalock SJ. Effects of media coverage of Women's Health Initiative study on attitudes and behavior of women receiving hormone replacement therapy. Am J Health Syst Pharm 2005 Jan 1;62(1):69–74.

7. "Pharma Drivers Provide Upside in 3Q Operating Results." Report on Wyeth prepared by Credit Suisse First Boston, October 20, 2004, p. 3.

8. Curhan GC et al, Lifetime nonnarcotic analgesic use and decline in renal function in women, Arch Intern Med 2004 Jul 26;164(14):1519–24.

9. Soberman J, Chafin CC, Weber KT. Aldosterone antagonists in congestive heart failure. Curr Opin Investig Drugs 2002 Jul;3(7):1024–8.

10. FDA Post Marketing Commitments, available at http://www.accessdata.fda.gov/scripts/cder/pmc/index.cfm.*

11. Innovation or Stagnation? Challenge and Opportunity on the Critical Path to New Medical Products, FDA White Paper, March, 2004..

12. White HD, Simes RJ, Anderson NE, et al. Pravastatin therapy and the risk of stroke. N Engl J Med 2000;343:317-326.

13. Schwartz GG, Olsson AG, Ezekowitz MD, et al. Effects of atorvastatin on recurrent ischemic events and acute coronary syndromes. The MIRACL study: a randomized controlled trial. JAMA 2001;285:1711-1718.

14. Jones PH, Hunninghake DB, Ferdinand KC. Effects of rosuvastatin versusatorvastatin, simvastatin, and pravastatin on non-high-density lipoprotein cholesterol, apolipoproteins, and lipid ratios in patients with hypercholesterolemia: additional results from the STELLAR trial. Clin Ther 2004 Sep 26;(9):1388-99, and McKenney JM, Jones PH, Adamczyk MA et al. Comparison of the efficacy of rosuvastatin versus atorvastatin, simvastatin and pravastatin in achieving lipid goals: results from the STELLAR trial. Current Medical Research and Opinions 2003;19(8):557–66.

15. Lewis EF, Moye LA. Predictors of late development of heart failure in stable survivors of myocardial infarction: the CARE study. J Am Coll Cardiol 2003 Oct 15;42(8):1446–53.

16. Shepherd J, Cobbe SM, Ford I et al. Prevention of coronary heart disease with pravastatin in men with hypercholesterolemia. West of Scotland Cornoary Prevention Study Group. N Engl J Med 1995 Nov 16;333(20):1301–7.

17. Pedersen, TR. Randomised trial of cholesterol lowering in 4444 patients with coronary heart disease: the Scandinavian Simvastatin Survival Study (4S). Atherosclerosis Supplements 2004;5:81–87.

18. Clearfield MDO, Downs JR. Air Force/Texas coronary atherosclerosis prevention study (AFCAPS/TexCAPS): Efficacy and tolerability of long-term treatment with lovastatin in women. Journal of Women's Health and Gender-Based Medicine 2001;10:971–81.

19. Heart Protection Study Collaborative Group. MRC/BHF Heart Protection Study of cholesterol lowering with simvastatin in 20,536 high-risk individuals: a randomised placebo-controlled trial. Lancet 2002;360:7–22.

20. Sever PS et al. Prevention of coronary and stroke events with atorvastatin in hypertensive patients who have average or lower-than-average cholesterol concentrations, in the Anglo-Scandinavian Cardiac Outcomes Trial--Lipid Lowering Arm (ASCOT-LLA): a multicentre randomised controlled trial. Lancet 2003 Apr 5;361(9364):1149–58.

21. Marshall G, McDougall C, Brady A and Fisher M. Should all diabetic patients receive a statin? Results from recent trials. Br J Cardiol 2004;11(6):455–60.

22. Smilde TJ, Trip MD, Wollersheim H, Kastelein JJP, Stalenhoef AFH. Rationale, design and baseline characteristics of a clinical trial comparing the effects of robust vs conventional cholesterol lowering and intima media

thickness in patients with familial hypercholesterolaemia: the Atorvastatin versus Simvastatin on Atherosclerosis Progression (ASAP) study. Clinical Drug Investagation 2000;20:67–79.

23. Ridker PM. Rosuvastatin in the primary prevention of cardiovascular disease among patients with low LDL cholesterol and elevated high sensitivity C-Reactive Protein (hsCRP): Rationale and design of the Jupiter Trial. Circulation 2003:108:2292–7.

24. Cannon CP, Braunwald E, McCabe CH. The Pravastatin or Atorvastatin evaluation and infection therapy—Thrombolysis in myocardial infarction 22 investigators: Intensive versus moderate lipid lowering with statins after acute coronary syndromes. N Engl J Med 2004;350:1495–1504.

25. Nissen SE, Tuzcu EM, Schoenhagen P et al. Effect of intensive compared with moderate lipid-lowering therapy on progression of coronary atherosclerosis: a randomised controlled trial. JAMA 2004;291:1071–80.

26. Koren MJ, Hunninghake DB. Clinical outcomes in managed-care patients with coronary heart disease treated aggressively in lipid-lowering disease management clinics: the alliance study. J Am Coll Cardiol 2004 Nov 2;44(9):1772–9.

27. DataEdge, the King of Research Statistics, Knows How Much You Charge for Research Studies, The Research Roundtable 1999 Sep;1(5).

28. Gilmartin, Raymond V. Remarks to the 2nd Annual National Congress on the Future of Genomics, Biotechnology and Pharmaceuticals in Medical Care, 17 Nov 2000. Available at: http://www.merck.com/newsroom/executive_speeches/.*

Note: All citations to websites listed in this book were verified in May of 2005.

3   What Makes It Different?

IN CONTRAST TO registration research, which involves a high-risk investment in products that may be many years away from approval, Phase IIIB and IV research represents an investment in products that are either already on the market and in use by the general public, or are at least expected to become available in the near future. Conducted in a different regulatory and commercial environment, strategic research is normally associated with greater design flexibility, increased cost sensitivity, and greater market awareness.

Design Flexibility

Pharmaceutical companies are reluctant to experiment with non-standard designs for their registration research given the conservative nature of the regulatory environment and its associated costs. Since marketing approval is a necessary milestone for the commercialization of any drug, the new drug application and review process represents a significant hurdle for new products. Companies want to put their absolute best foot forward during this process to minimize potential approval delays and restrictions that could result if they followed non-standard approaches to clinical research.

The pharmaceutical industry has made a science of understanding how regulators think during the approval process. This understanding represents a familiarity with all written regulatory requirements as well as knowledge of how these written requirements have been interpreted in practice. In much the same way as written legislation is given depth through a history of judicial interpretation, the filing strategy for a new product gets more complex as more regulatory advisories and decisions further define the approval process—adding ongoing costs to the drug development process.

THE INCREASING COST OF NEW DRUG APPROVAL

Although pharmaceutical research and development spending has increased steadily over the past two decades, the number of new drugs approved has tended to trend downward since 1997. Behind this trend is the increasing average cost of bringing a drug to market.[1]

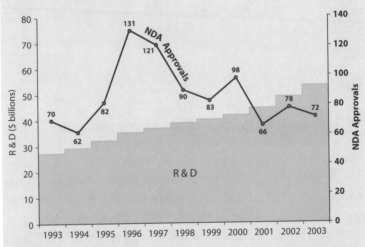

FIGURE 3. Global Pharmaceutical R&D spending in billions of dollars (shaded) versus the number of NDA approvals granted by the FDA (line).

Armed with experience in the regulatory decision-making process, pharmaceutical companies do not embark on the long and expensive drug development process only to skim the bar at the time of NDA submission. With up to $800 million for Phase I–III research at stake, companies feel that they have little to gain and much to lose by deviating from traditional approaches to study design, monitoring, data collection, and endpoint analysis during registration research. If the company cannot afford to take the most risk-averse approach on the basis of the drug's expected commercial potential, it will shelve the molecule and work on another.

Once companies receive a favorable response to their NDA submission, however, they can be less conservative in the research they support. No longer fearing a loss of their earlier investment on a regulatory technicality, companies can now design studies based on good clinical practice and scientific imagination rather than on regulatory expectations. The relative freedom of strategic research explains why innovative designs, processes, and technologies have been more broadly adopted in Phases IIIB and IV, and why efficiencies emerging from these new approaches have had a very limited impact on the increasing cost of drug development associated with Phases I–III. The various study designs that can be valuable after submission of the NDA are described in detail in chapter four.

DIFFERENT OPERATIONAL ALTERNATIVES

Just as variation from the randomized controlled trial format is more common in Phases IIIB and IV than in registration research, companies are also more receptive to different operational approaches when conducting strategic research. Because products are now available in the real world, it is possible to do naturalistic studies. It is also possible to study products for indefinite periods of time. In addition, since operational processes can be adapted to reflect an increased confidence in the effectiveness and safety of a drug after pivotal trials are completed, sponsors are turning to creative methods such as remote monitoring and direct-from-patient data collection to conduct their studies more efficiently.

For example, active surveillance studies are frequently performed to evaluate the safety of products in the post-marketing period. To ensure that these programs encourage maximum patient enrollment and avoid selection bias, it has become common for safety surveillance programs to seek a waiver of informed patient consent from ethics committees or IRBs. This waiver is usually granted on the basis that patients are not subject to any additional risks as a result of a naturalistic study protocol, and privacy is protected by the appropriate de-identification of data.

Cost Sensitivity

Registration research is usually funded from the consolidated R&D budget as a cost of conducting business. Phase IIIB and IV research, in contrast, is most often funded from an annual brand budget and internally accounted for as a cost of goods sold. Manufacturers often perceive this research as a voluntary investment in a brand, which therefore competes for funding with other activities such as medical education and communications, advertising, sales teams, and sponsorships.* This is usually the case even when the responsibility for designing and managing clinical research is appropriately separated from a company's marketing function. Because these competing activities are often relatively short and cheap, strategic research is under greater pressure than

---

*Even though regulators have increasingly demanded additional post-marketing studies as a condition of approval, there have been few repercussions for the many companies that have not yet fully met, or even commenced, their regulatory commitments.

registration research to prove itself valuable, timely, and reasonably priced while remaining in compliance with good clinical practice.

Once approved, most products will generate considerable return with no additional research investment. As a result, Phase IIIB and IV research is funded on a project-by-project basis with an emphasis on maximizing the value of each study to the company. Companies ask themselves, "How much can I gain if I do this study?" and "How much could I lose if I don't do it?" thus regularly balancing their opportunities and public health responsibilities against cost and risk.

Invariably, by competing with other non-research activities for funding, and by requiring project-by-project justification for investment, Phase IIIB and IV research programs are much more cost sensitive than is registration research. For this reason, strategic research programs have needed to adopt more creative study designs and cost-effective operational approaches, such as electronic data collection, centralized project coordination, remote monitoring services, direct-from-consumer data collection, and offshore data processing.

DOING RESEARCH ON A BRAND BUDGET

A cardiovascular study conducted for registration purposes cost a major pharmaceutical company almost $6 million, although it involved fewer than 500 patients and only 25 sites. The company reproduced the study, using the same number of patients and sites but with a different patient population for just under $1 million. Faced with a limited budget for the brand, and no longer constrained by regulatory requirements, the pharmaceutical sponsor willingly considered alternative approaches to site selection, site monitoring, and data capture, which resulted in significant cost savings.

Market Awareness

Conducted in parallel with a flurry of commercial activities—advertising, product detailing, medical education, conferences, and speaker tours—effective execution of Phase IIIB and IV research demands an intimate understanding of the commercial side of the pharmaceutical business. Phase IIIB and IV research involves brands, not just drugs, and needs to be intimately coordinated within a much bigger picture of business activity.

In earlier phase studies, the company is researching a molecule; somewhere between discovery and launch that molecule becomes a brand. Clinical researchers who worked with the molecule UK-92480 faced different challenges and market expectations than those working with Viagra, as the molecule is known today.

Unlike registration research, Phase IIIB and IV research is subject to promotional laws and restrictions that apply to all business activities involving marketed products. In addition, a whole new set of pharmaco-vigilance reporting responsibilities also apply. Whereas earlier clinical research was the only business activity involving a product, any ongoing research conducted after regulatory filing becomes just a small part of a much bigger brand support machine—tolerated by commercial operations on the basis that its execution does not significantly interfere with them. Understanding the roles of investigators, key opinion leaders, medical directors, sales representatives, nurse advisors, sales managers, and brand managers—some of whom may have little or no clinical research experience—is critical to the success of working within a much bigger team, and ultimately to the success of any research activities.

Conclusion

Phase IIIB and IV research represents an upside opportunity for products that are either already on the market or are expected to generate revenue in the near future. As a result, pharmaceutical companies are more open to deviating from traditional approaches to clinical research than when product approval remains at risk. In addition, shorter term return on investment expectations, requirement for greater commercial sensitivity, and greater competition with non-research activities for funding creates demand for cost effectiveness, design flexibility, and market awareness not normally associated with registration research.

References

1. NDA data appears on www.fda.gov/cder/rdmt/pstable.htm. Pharmaceutical R&D data is from CMR International 2004 R&D Factbook, Center for Medicines Research International (2004). www.cmr.org.*

Note: All citations to websites listed in this book were verified in May of 2005.

II Fundamentals of Strategic Research

4 Design Possibilities

RANDOMIZED CONTROLLED TRIALS (RCTs) represent the gold standard for testing a clinical hypothesis. Since most regulators demand hard evidence in support of new drug applications, and since most pharmaceutical companies try to follow the lowest risk path to product approval, it is not surprising that most Phase II and III studies follow this design.

Although most sponsors favor RCT designs for their registration trials, they frequently choose other approaches for their Phase IIIB and IV studies to save time, minimize cost and avoid ethical challenges associated with conducting experimental treatment protocols in patients. Choosing an appropriate design often means balancing the need for rigorous scientific proof against a need for timely information, or against the morality of assigning patients to receive treatments of significantly different risk or efficacy. For example, it would be unethical to measure the effect of a new treatment on healthcare utilization by asking one group to take the new product and another group to use the incumbent market leader which has already been proven clinically inferior in earlier stage studies.

This chapter briefly describes different study designs commonly used in Phase IIIB and IV research. It begins with a discussion of randomized controlled trials and different options for minimizing reporting bias, and then turns to a discussion of non-experimental approaches to clinical research using retrospective, cross-sectional and prospective observational study designs. Those wanting more details are encouraged to seek further information from a specialist text on clinical trials design, biostatistics, or epidemiology.[1]

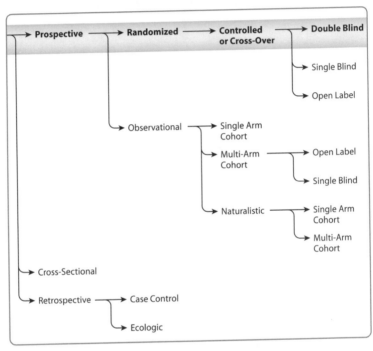

FIGURE 4. A CLINICAL TRIAL TAXONOMY. Phase IIIB and IV researchers can choose from a wide variety of study designs, balancing the need for statistical strength offered by randomized, double blind, controlled trials against the speed, simplicity, cost, and ethical benefits of other approaches.

Randomized Controlled Studies

Patients participating in RCTs are randomly assigned to one of several treatment groups. This process of "randomization", first proposed by Sir Ronald A. Fisher in 1919, allows researchers to establish a control experiment by ensuring that all variables except for the treatment received are kept roughly constant between patient groups. Doing so increases the chance that different outcomes observed between the groups can be attributed to the different treatments that they received.

To minimize the effect of measurement and reporting bias on study results, some studies require that neither the patient nor the investigator know which treatment the patient is receiving. This process, known as double-blinding, increases the statistical strength of a study and is the most highly regarded method for conducting randomized clinical research but can be unpopular with research naive physicians and patients who are not comfortable with losing control over treatment decisions. In addition, sponsors can face significant delays and costs associated with manufacturing treatment formulations that must be indistinguishable from each other for double-blinding to work. Sometimes researchers compromise by allowing the physician (but not the patient) to know what treatment the patient is receiving, a process known as single-blinding. Single-blinding is often used to evaluate surgical interventions or drugs that need frequent dose titration since it is not possible for the investigator to avoid knowing what treatments are being used.

In contrast, open-label studies allow both patients and physicians to know which treatment each patient is receiving — introducing the possibility of reporting bias but minimizing the cost and timeline for obtaining study results and expanding the number of physicians that might be interested in participating in the research. Patients and their physicians usually feel more comfortable knowing what drugs they are taking, and it is easier for sponsors to use their normal supply of drug in the trial.

After the clinical efficacy of a new medicine has been proven in Phase II and III studies, many physicians want to know about the net effectiveness and safety of the product — including any effect that its packaging, formulation, and brand placebo effect may have on its tolerability, usability, and compliance. Understanding that a treatment is more than just a molecule, many physicians value health outcomes demonstrated through open-label research because it attempts to characterize the value of a product when used as it would be in the real world. Wherever possible, open-label randomized studies attempt to avoid reporting bias by using objective machine measurable endpoints, such as total cholesterol, temperature, body mass index, or blood pressure. To avoid the possibility of test results feeding back to influence treatment, many researchers choose to keep patients and their physicians blind to the results of their individual endpoint measures — creating what is popularly referred to as the PROBE (prospective, randomized, observational blinded endpoints) design.

THE PROBE DESIGN

The prospective, randomized, open, blinded endpoints (PROBE) design has become popular for research involving large numbers of patients or comparison of treatments with very different routes of administration, both of which make double-blind trials very complex and costly. PROBE designs have been well established in cardiovascular research, most particularly in hypertension studies, following the success of the ASCOT trial, which randomized over 19,000 patients to one of two different open-label antihypertensive treatment programs. The open-label design was necessary in this case for three reasons: (1) because physicians were required to tightly control blood pressure through frequent dose titration (hard to do if the physician does not know which drugs they have to titrate), (2) because physicians were required to closely monitor for electrolyte disturbances in patients receiving diuretic treatment, and (3) because the large study size required that study designers focus on reducing workload burden and cost.[2]

Subsequent meta-analyses of both PROBE and double-blind placebo-controlled hypertension studies have demonstrated the statistical equivalence of their results, and provided validity of the PROBE design as a powerful research alternative.[3]

Observational Methodologies

Randomized studies involve the setup of an experiment to compare treatment outcomes between different patient groups with patient treatment dictated by a study protocol rather than a physician's standard of care. Although an RCT represents the gold standard for testing a clinical hypothesis, there are many different non-experimental study designs that can still yield valuable clinical information much more quickly, straightforwardly, cheaply—and sometimes more ethically—than this experimental approach.

These non-experimental designs, also known collectively as observational studies, can be retrospective (using data that has already been captured), cross-sectional (capturing patient data at one point in time), and prospective (enrolling and tracking patients over time). Following is a brief discussion of each approach, with case examples to illustrate the role of these different study designs in the clinical research process.

Retrospective Studies

Retrospective studies use historical data to populate a study database; the most common example, the chart review, captures data from patient files. Retrospective studies are much cheaper than prospective or cross-sectional studies, which typically involve the prospective enrollment and consent of patients. Many retrospective studies simply require that sites transpose de-identified summary data from their existing files into a study database for analysis, in most cases avoiding lengthy administrative processes. Retrospective studies can be completed even more quickly if researchers choose to use claims databases or existing clinical registries to support ongoing data analyses.

Because retrospective studies usually involve different data points collected at multiple points in time for each patient, they are recognized as being more effective at inferring causality than a cross-sectional study but are frequently challenged by critics who can only be satisfied by RCT data. On August 25, 2004, Dr. David Graham presented the results of an FDA-funded retrospective analysis of Kaiser Permanente health record claims. The highly publicized study suggested that patients receiving Merck's Vioxx treatment had experienced a significantly greater rate of cardiovascular events than those receiving older non-steroidal agents. Not surprisingly, even though the media reaction to this data was intense, many industry analysts and key opinion leaders initially responded cautiously to this study because Graham's analysis was not an RCT.

Graham's announcement of his retrospective Kaiser Permanente data analysis provides an excellent example of how these studies can establish interesting hypotheses to direct further research; less than 14 days later, following an analysis of data from their own randomized Vioxx studies, Merck decided the link between Vioxx and cardiovascular risk had sufficient scientific validity and announced the biggest global product recall in history.

Case-control design. The case-control design involves identifying patients with a given health outcome ("cases") and those without the outcome ("controls"), and then looking back in time to compare the frequency of an exposure in the case group to the control group. The case-control design is commonly used to study rare health outcomes and is sometimes the only ethical way to investigate an association.

CASE-CONTROL CASE STUDY

To identify risk factors for intrauterine fetal death (IUFD), researchers from Nottingham City Hospital compared data from 161 singleton stillbirth pregnancies that occurred between 1991 and 1997 with data from 499 randomly selected live births that occurred during the same period.[4] The study identified several factors as being positively associated with IUFD—small size for gestational age, maternal body mass index, maternal age, and maternal type O blood group—but revealed no association between stillbirth rate and maternal ethnicity, Rhesus status, fetal sex, or smoking.

Ecological design. An alternative retrospective approach, population-based rather than individual-subject based, involves aggregating patient data at investigational sites and then transmitting only a summary of this data back to the study center for analysis. In most regions, the process of aggregation at a group level avoids privacy issues. For example, an investigator may wish to study the mortality rate associated with different types of chemotherapy treatment. Rather than asking five oncology centers to submit patient-level data, the investigator may simply ask each center to provide high-level data regarding the number of patients being treated with different chemotherapy programs and the mortality rate associated with each group.

While retrospective studies are relatively quick and cheap to implement, the quality and completeness of data collection is dependent upon the quality and appropriateness of data recorded in the medical history or other data repositories. It is often impossible to go back and query data, and even then data points are limited to those recorded during the standard consultation process. Retrospective research concludes with many values still missing and data queries unresolved.

Cross-Sectional Studies

Cross-sectional studies, as their name suggests, involve collection of data from a patient at a single point in time. Usually, cross-sectional studies try to enroll patients over a short period of time to prevent time lapse over the data collection period from influencing results. For instance, an allergy study will yield lower severity scores if patient enrollment spans beyond spring.

Cross-sectional studies represent a cheaper and quicker way to obtain data than prospective research while offering more control over question design and data completeness than a retrospective approach. Cross-sectional study designs are most commonly used for determining prevalence (the number of cases in a population at a given point in time), but they can be used to identify possible associations without a long trial. Sometimes the inference of causality by a cross-sectional study is sufficient to change a clinical behavior. For example, the mechanism of action for a new painkiller may suggest a theoretical gastrointestinal benefit. A cross-sectional study of patients receiving painkillers may reveal that gastric pain is less prevalent in patients receiving this new drug than in those receiving other drugs on the market. While this is clearly not proof of its relative safety, these results may be enough to make many prescribers preferentially prescribe the new drug to patients with gastrointestinal irritability.

CROSS-SECTIONAL CASE STUDY

Interested in understanding more about the functional disability of rheumatoid arthritis, researchers from Norway conducted a cross-sectional study of 706 European patients who had had rheumatoid arthritis for at least four years.[5] They assessed the functional disability of each patient at a point in time and collected information regarding possible risk factors and markers for disease activity. The study demonstrated that female sex, high erythrocyte sedimentation rate (ESR), and disease duration strongly and independently correlated with functional disability, while the presence of rheumatoid factor, joint damage as observed on X-ray, increasing age, and education did not. The results of this study have helped physicians recognize that women are at particularly high risk of disability even in the early stages of the disease, which has justified more aggressive approaches to early treatment.

Prospective Observational Studies

A prospective observational study, also known as a prospective cohort study, is one that simply monitors a group (or cohort) of patients over time without mandating any treatment intervention. Most industry references to "observational research" usually relate to this prospective approach, where the decision to treat is the physician's alone and any treatment prescribed during the study would have been considered by the physician whether or not the patient was a study participant. Observational studies can involve a schedule of follow-up visits and tests that are not part of usual clinical practice, and sometimes involve blinding the patient but obviously not their treating physician, to the treatment they receive.

These studies—particularly for approved products—present little risk to patients since they allow the treating physician to remain in control of all treatment decisions. As a result, they require less monitoring activity (and therefore less cost) than an RCT to ensure data quality and patient safety, and patient recruitment is much easier. Prospective observational studies often represent a compromise for sponsors who require very large amounts of high quality targeted data not available through other sources, but who cannot justify the cost or timeline associated with conducting an RCT.

Naturalistic Designs

A naturalistic (or actual use) study is a special case of a prospective observational study that not only avoids mandating any treatment intervention but also avoids scheduling non-standard visits, examinations, or investigations that are not otherwise performed in routine practice. People often mistakenly use the term "naturalistic" to describe studies that are actually observational. A naturalistic study, by definition, is always observational; an observational study is not always naturalistic.

Sponsors perform naturalistic studies when it is important that the conduct of a study itself should not influence patient care patterns and treatment outcomes. A study that offers free study drug is not naturalistic, since patients may be more compliant and less likely to discontinue treatment than if they purchased drug through a formulary. A study that involves more visits than those normally associated with routine patient care is not naturalistic, since the increased frequency of review may change the way a physician treats patients. Similarly, a study that mandates particular tests is not naturalistic, since the results of tests performed outside naturalistic practice may influence patient care. Would a physician ignore a high cholesterol result obtained through a clinical trial even if the patient were not otherwise scheduled for a cholesterol test for another six months?

NATURALISTIC CASE STUDY
Sometimes the effectiveness of a treatment is dependent upon a much wider range of factors than molecular efficacy alone. This is particularly so in the case of dementia, where the quality of non-medical patient care can have a significant effect on patient health outcomes and the burden the disease places on families. To assess the impact of Reminyl (galantamine) on behavioral disturbances and associated caregiver burden when used under naturalistic conditions, investigators from Switzerland tracked the outcomes of 124 patients initiated on

the treatment. The study demonstrated significantly reduced behavioral disturbances in this population after three months and a measurable reduction in caregiver burden. For primary care physicians who are managing the health and stress of caregivers as well as patients, this data is likely to be more influential as a guide to treatment than RCT results supporting a small clinical effect on cognitive function.[6]

Parallel-Cohort Designs

Whereas most prospective observational studies track clinical outcomes for a single treatment group, it is occasionally useful to follow multiple treatment groups, or cohorts, in parallel. By comparing outcomes from two different groups, researchers can use an observational approach to answer complex clinical questions.

Using tight inclusion/exclusion criteria to ensure that confounding characteristics are equally balanced between study groups, researchers can establish a prospective observational study that approximates a randomized design. For example, an observational protocol may ask a physician to enroll the first three healthy males, aged 30–35, receiving drug X, and the first three healthy males with the same clinical characteristics taking drug Y. As long as both populations have similar characteristics at the time of analysis (homogeneity generally improves as study samples increase), comparative analysis through direct comparison or case matching may be possible. Researchers can apply a number of statistical techniques to maximize the significance of conclusions drawn.

Hybrid Studies

Many strategic research studies patch together multiple design approaches, attempting to capitalize on the speed, cost-efficiency, and empirical strength of different designs by combining them within a research program. Such approaches include mixing cross-sectional designs with retrospective data capture, thereby approximating a prospective observational approach without the time delay. Other approaches include running a simple prospective study across a large number of sites in parallel with a set of smaller, more complex randomized controlled sub-studies at a subset of sites. Mixing designs in this manner can be cost effective and powerful but can also introduce risk to the analytical integrity of the project if not conducted by individuals with experience in study design.

Hybrid Case Study

Establishing the effectiveness of a treatment in reducing patient mortality or morbidity can be time consuming when the therapy is used to prevent illness rather than to treat disease. Sometimes it is necessary to follow patients for five to ten years before the real impact of a treatment can be established. One company, keen to rapidly obtain this data in support of their preventative cardiovascular treatment, commenced a hybrid study including both retrospective and prospective components. Primary care physicians were asked to identify a pool of patients who had already received at least three years of treatment with the active drug, as well as a much larger secondary pool of patients who had received treatment with a competitive product during the same period. A case matching process was undertaken based on patient characteristics at the time that therapy was originally initiated. Prospective follow-up of clinical markers and patient outcomes is now taking place over a two-year period, with regular comparative analysis to detect deviation in survival outcomes. By taking this approach, the sponsor is likely to generate strong data in support of their product years before results from their long-term RCT are available.

Conclusion

The relative benefits and costs of different clinical trial designs available to the researcher in Phase IIIB and IV are summarized in the tables below, including their capacity to answer a range of questions (breadth).

TO IDENTIFY TRENDS (e.g. How should drug X best be prescribed?)		Type of Trial	Time	Cost	Breadth
	QUICKLY (But less robust)	Cross-Sectional	2-6m	$0.5-2m	HIGH
	ROBUSTLY (But less quickly)	Prospective Observational Multi-Arm	12-18m	$1-5m	HIGH
	COMPROMISE	Prospective Observational Single-Arm	6-18m	$0.5-5m	HIGH

TO TEST A HYPOTHESIS (e.g. Drug X is equally effective at 40 and 80mg doses)		Type of Trial	Time	Cost	Breadth
	WITH CONCLUSIVE PROOF	Randomized Control (RCT)	1-3 yrs	$1-20m	LOW
	WITH STRONG PROOF	Retrospective Case Control	0-6m	$0.2-1m	LOW
	... BUT DON'T HAVE THE DATASET	Prospective Observational	6-18m	$0.5-5m	HIGH
	... AND DON'T HAVE THE TIME	Cross-Sectional	2-6m	$0.5-2m	HIGH

Strategic research can benefit from the wide variety of design options available to investigators. While Phase IIIB and IV researchers frequently use the most rigorous randomized, controlled, double blind designs, they also commonly use observational studies and open-label designs. These are often more compatible with normal clinical workflow and may provide sufficiently relevant data more quickly, easily, and cheaply than would be possible taking a randomized double-blind controlled trial approach.

References

1. See Friedman, LM, Fruberg, CD. Fundamentals of Clinical Trials, 3rd ed. (Springer: 1999) and Piantadosi, S. Clinical Trials: A Methodologic Perspective, BK&Disk ed. (Wiley-Interscience: 1977).

2. Sever et al, Rationale, design, methods and baseline demography of participants of the Anglo-Scandinavian Cardiac Outcomes Trial. J Hypertens. June 2001;19(6): 1139–47.

3. Smith et al. Prospective, randomized, open-label, blinded-endpoint (PROBE) designed trials yield the same results as double-blind, placebo-controlled trials with respect to ABPM measurements. J Hypertens July 2003;21(7): 1291–8.

4. Efkarpidis et al. Case-control study of factors associated with intrauterine fetal deaths. Medscape General Medicine 2004;6(2), available at http://www.medscape.com/viewarticle/476183.*

5. Smedstad et al. Correlates of functional disability in early rheumatoid arthritis: a cross-sectional study of 706 patients in four European countries. Br J Rheumatol. 1996 Aug;35(8):746–51.

6. Monsch et al. Effects of galantamine on behavioural and psychological disturbances and caregiver burden in patients with Alzheimer's disease. Curr Med Res Opin 2004;20(6): 931–84.

*Note: All citations to websites listed in this book were verified in May of 2005.

5

Regulatory Considerations

A NUMBER OF DIFFERENT public agencies have an interest in the pharmaceutical industry, including those responsible for verifying whether new treatments are safe and effective, those charged with monitoring promotional practices, and those overseeing public health services and government insurance programs.

Although the industry has always taken a more flexible approach toward Phase IIIB and IV research than to registration research, as we will see in the first section of this chapter, it would be a mistake to think of strategic research as being unregulated and lawless. In fact, in addition to principles of good clinical practice, strategic research is subject to its own unique laws (many enforced by significant financial and criminal penalties) that vary significantly from country to country and primarily relate to off-label promotion, product supply, financial inducement, and patient privacy.

Clearing the Bar

The International Conference for Harmonization: Good Clinical Practice (ICH-GCP) established a minimum standard for clinical research in May 1996. Although most countries recognize ICH-GCP as the international ethical and scientific quality standard for the conduct and reporting of trials that involve the participation of human subjects, practical interpretation of this standard has been subject to local regulatory debate since it was finalized. Most regulators have their own ideas about what ICH-GCP actually means in practice, but local interpretations are united in their conservative attitude towards applying ICH-GCP to registration research. This consistency breaks down in Phases IIIB and IV, however, with regional differences so great that a study design demanded as a condition of approval by one country may be illegal to conduct in another.

In the United States the FDA has developed volumes of notifications and advisories that expand on these guidelines. Other nations have their own interpretations of the guidelines: the European Union has adopted the European Clinical Trials Directive (EU-CTD) and its European Medicines Evaluation Agency (EMEA) is continually expanding on this directive; Australia has adopted the National Health & Medical Research Council's Guidelines for Good Clinical Research Practice (GCRP); and Japan is still subject to the idiosyncracies of the Pharmaceutical Affairs Law despite adopting ICH-GCP in the late 1990s.

Although ICH-GCP sets a minimum standard for the conduct of clinical studies, most sponsors have created their own standard operating procedures (SOPs) that not only meet the standards set by GCP but also attempt to address more detailed local standards and FDA/EMEA precedents established over the past 25 years. In an attempt to address these different standards and interpretations, most corporate SOPs set a much higher bar than ICH-GCP or the EU-CTD.

The gap between a sponsor's processes and those established by ICH-GCP represent the additional lengths to which a sponsor is willing to go to minimize the risk of a technical rejection of submission data. It is not unusual for registration studies to be loaded with $10 million to $20 million of additional activity not explicitly required by regulatory agencies. Of the few companies that have attempted a less conservative approach, most have learned the hard way that taking risks with a new drug application is simply not worth it.

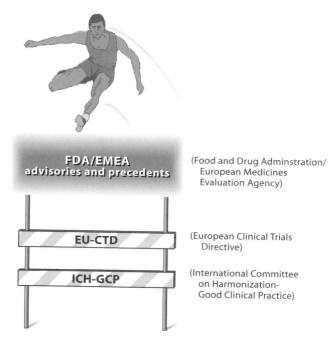

FDA/EMEA advisories and precedents
(Food and Drug Adminstration/ European Medicines Evaluation Agency)

EU-CTD
(European Clinical Trials Directive)

ICH-GCP
(International Committee on Harmonization- Good Clinical Practice)

FIGURE 5.1 In Phase I–III trials, pharmaceutical manufacturers aim high to clear regulatory hurdles to ensure that their studies address local regulatory interpretations and precedents that could result in approval delays. But many companies are beginning to establish Phase IIIB/IV specific SOPs that address GCP but avoid unnecessary process once the regulatory hurdle of product approval has been overcome.

Since many of these costly additional procedures do little to protect patient safety or data quality, many sponsors are more comfortable taking a more practical view of ICH-GCP once the regulatory hurdle of product approval has been overcome. Recognizing that process for process sake is both expensive and a poor use of physicians' time, many pharmaceutical companies are establishing Phase IIIB and IV SOPs that are designed to comfortably address the spirit of the ICH-GCP guidance while providing much greater latitude for study design and cost containment.

Many people incorrectly assume that a "Phase IIIB/IV" approach must be less clinically robust. This is not so. It simply reflects an understanding that ICH-GCP allows for context-sensitive research practices. Some Phase IIIB and IV studies may need exactly the same level of administrative due diligence applied as do registration activities, but not all. Inappropriately applied processes can increase the burden of strategic research to patients and investigators, sometimes jeopardizing research feasibility without improving clinical robustness.

CLINICAL TRIAL MONITORING

Most regulators have an expectation that studies conducted in support of marketing authorization are subject to 100 percent source-data verification performed through frequent on-site monitoring visits. ICH-GCP taken on its own, however, does not insist upon this. Rather it allows for various forms of monitoring depending on the study being conducted.

"The determination of the extent, and nature of monitoring should be based on considerations such as the objective, purpose, design, complexity, blinding, size and endpoints of the trial. In general there is a need for on-site monitoring, before, during and after the trial; however ... central monitoring in conjunction with procedures such as investigators' training and meetings and extensive written guidance can assure appropriate conduct of the trial in accordance with GCP. Statistically controlled sampling may be an acceptable for selecting the data to be verified ..." (ICH-GCP).[1]

Although most companies do not take advantage of this freedom to choose a monitoring method during registration trials, a number of large companies are starting to explore processes in strategic research such as computerized monitoring (of electronic data) and structured remote telephone monitoring that can significantly reduce the frequency and cost of on-site visits while maintaining data quality and protocol compliance.

Promotional Regulations

Phase IIIB and IV research activity can benefit from greater operational design opportunities (as explained in the previous chapter) and a more practical interpretation of ICH-GCP than earlier phase clinical trials, but this research can also be subject to a range of geography-specific regulatory considerations not applicable in earlier phases. Over the past 25 years, most countries have introduced regulations governing the sales and marketing of pharmaceutical products. These regulations cover a wide range of matters, including justification of claims, off-label prescribing, medical education, and potential conflict of interest by companies in their interactions with physicians.

Most importantly, because strategic research is conducted in parallel with intense promotional activity, the research is subject to the same promotional regulations that apply to the sponsor's sales and marketing activities. Studies must be designed with sufficient rigor to avoid even appearing to encourage off-label prescribing or to perpetuate false claims. The involvement of sales representatives can obviously introduce risks; not so clear is that a CRA calling upon physicians during this period must also be aware of what they can and cannot say in regard to promotional regulations. Most regulatory environments do not make a distinction between these two types of sponsor representatives. A CRA must operate within the same compliance boundaries as a sales representative, and these boundaries are often much stricter once a product is on the market.

Product Supply

Many countries have different rules regarding the supply of investigational product during different phases of clinical research. The study sponsor almost always supplies pre-approval investigational product; post-marketing studies are often conducted using the commercially available product. This is particularly common when performing naturalistic studies: where the supply of study drug may influence product compliance and persistency; where maintaining a wide product inventory for naturalistic dose titration is not practical; or when an investigational product is to be evaluated against naturalistic "standard care."

A number of countries, including Germany, attempt to prevent sponsors' using reimbursed field stock to support Phase IV research, even for post-marketing safety surveillance activities that require very large patient numbers.

Financial Inducement

Some countries have taken a hard-line approach to studies that directly influence prescribing of state-reimbursed medication through the conduct of the study. The United States, for example, has applied the Anti-kickback statute, which likens any payment to an investigator for the purpose of inducing the prescription of federal or state reimbursed product, to bribery of a government official in anticipation of financial gain, an offense with significant civil and criminal penalties.

Seeding studies, once popular in the United States, have been directly targeted by these anti-kickback measures (see the appendix). These studies, frequently associated with large numbers of investigators and sites, involve paying physicians sums of money to initiate patients on reimbursed product while only asking them to collect nominal information. Unfortunately, applying anti-kickback laws to studies has affected many legitimate study

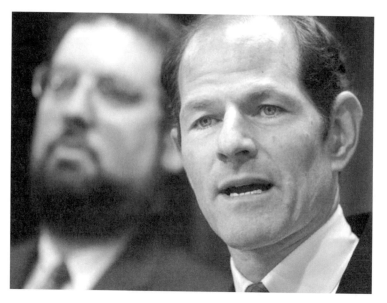

FIGURE 5.2 Post-marketing research practices are under increasing scrutiny by regulators, politicians, and community activists around the world. New York Attorney General Eliot Spitzer has taken an interest in Phase IIIB and IV trials examining the use of anti-depressants in children.

designs and is beginning to affect patient access to medication in expanded access programs and open-label extension phases.*

Not all regions take this hard-line approach, however, as indicated by the findings of a 2001 report by the Netherlands Health Care Inspectorate. This report, which involved an analysis of corporate marketing plans, estimated spending on seeding studies to exceed 20 percent of annual marketing budgets for Netherlands-based pharmaceutical companies. Although the European Council Directive 92/28/EEC has prohibited pharmaceutical companies from using direct or indirect financial inducements to influence prescription practices since 1992, lack of enforcement has allowed seeding studies to remain a common part of the marketing land-

---

*These are added to Phase III and IIIB studies so that patients can continue to benefit from treatment until a product is finally approved.

scape in many European countries.[2]

Privacy

Over the past five years, legislatures have taken a range of measures to protect individual privacy in an age of increasing data collection and sharing. Some of these measures have been specifically addressed in the Health Insurance Portability and Accountability Act of 1996 (HIPAA) in the United States and the European Union Privacy Directive. These measures have been designed to target all healthcare interactions, and clinical research activities must operate in compliance with them. Differences in privacy legislation across countries require differences in the study start-up process, patient consent activities and data collection and processing, thus making it complex when data must cross borders either for off-shore entry or for management in a centralized database.

Conclusion

In meeting regulatory requirements, there are more gray areas in the practice of strategic research than in registration research. There is greater freedom to design a range of clinical studies and less fear of not meeting a regulatory bar. But strategic research is no regulatory panacea. There is a wider field for opportunity, but it is filled with landmines in new locations because the product is simultaneously in commercial distribution and research settings.

References

1. ICH-GCP document, draft revised 2004-07-02. Workstream 4: Trial Management and Monitoring, part C) Monitoring Procedures. Available at http://www.ct-toolkit.ac.uk/_db/_documents/Trial_MP.pdf*

2. Marketing plans for medicinal products available on prescription only: the current situation, Health Care Inspectorate, Netherlands, July 2001, second revised edition.

*Note: All citations to websites listed in this book were verified in May of 2005.

6 Maximizing Value

LARGE PHARMACEUTICAL COMPANIES are frustrated by the lack of impact from Phase IIIB and IV research, especially given the amount of money they spend in this area. To address this problem, brand team members need to understand that the impact and value of a Phase IIIB or IV study is measured not only by the statistical significance of its results but by a combination of factors that include the scientific immediacy of the research to patients and physicians and—even more importantly—the timing of its conduct. A successful strategic research plan involves having what you need to say when you need to say it, and is most effective when you keep goals focused, keep studies simple, and communicate both internally and externally.

Plan Ahead

The culture of the pharmaceutical industry is not conducive to rapid decision-making. The most effective companies recognize that the process of developing a research strategy, creating a protocol, obtaining necessary internal approvals, and securing funding is a long and slow process that can delay a response to a market opportunity or crisis. To address these delays, brand teams develop a research wish list by identifying:

· · · · ·

- weaknesses in their existing data that could compromise their ability to differentiate their products effectively,

- opportunities to supplement existing data in support of the value of their product,

- and "safety net" data that could be useful in the event of a product or competitive crisis.

Researchers develop a range of research protocol synopses around this wish list and establish budgets, timeframes, and priorities for each opportunity. To maximize the value of their research investment, they must consider whether multiple objectives can be addressed within one study or conversely whether multiple studies could synergistically support an objective.

By proactively developing a portfolio of possible research protocols (not all will be funded) in anticipation of the brand teams needs, companies can react to market changes three to six months faster than their competitors. Having these procedures in place allows a company to kick off pre-approved protocols quickly, improving its chances of producing the right data at the right time.

RAPID RESPONSE DEMONSTRATES COMMITMENT TO SAFETY

In 2002, Johnson & Johnson (J&J) faced growing concern over the safety of their blockbuster treatment for anemia, Eprex (erythropoietin alfa). Regulators were growing concerned by a slow but significant increase in the incidence of Pure Red Cell Aplasia (PRCA), a rare adverse event, among patients receiving Eprex by subcutaneous injection. Although the cause of increasing PRCA was not known at the time, J&J reacted rapidly by initiating an Urgent Safety Restriction (USR) to ensure intravenous administration of the medicine while, at the same time, announcing an extensive epidemiological study of patients receiving erythropoietin treatment. The study's goals were to better understand risk factors for PRCA development, to monitor and confirm the safety of intravenous administration, and to ensure that the USR was effective in reducing Eprex's subcutaneous use. Facing stiff competition from a new erythropoietin drug manufactured by Amgen, J&J's rapid actions not only reaffirmed the company's commitment to safety, but prevented a broader product restriction that could have quickly cost J&J a sizeable part of their $1.1 billion Eprex franchise.[1]

Know Your Goals

Strategic research is associated with greater latitude in protocol design than registration research and it is also used to answer many different questions than the earlier phase research. These expanded means and goals make it possible for studies to proceed without clearly defined research aims or endpoints, causing many projects to fall flat on value because of a lack of clarity and focus in their original design. Just because it is possible to conduct studies that span a broad range of objectives in Phase IIIB and IV does not mean that you should.

Designing strategic research activities should start with how you want to use the data, when you want to use it, and to whom it needs to be addressed.

The design of a Phase IIIB and IV study is equally influenced by its scientific objectives and by the need for information due to market context. Failure to clearly identify a study's scientific goals and its target audience can result in the execution of inappropriately designed studies and the underachievement of research potential. Many companies commence "catch all" studies on the basis that valuable data may turn up. Unfortunately, this is almost never the case.

Keep It Simple

As well as remaining focused on the goals of a Phase IIIB or IV study, it is equally important to minimize the operational complexity of each project. Address different objectives through multiple simple protocols that are coordinated as a program of parallel studies and/or sub studies rather than as a single complex protocol. Every unnecessary protocol complexity places the smooth execution of a study at risk, and every extraneous data point collected increases disclosure risks associated with holding data that may not be exhaustively analyzed.

Protecting the simplicity of a study increases the chance that researchers can control its timing and manage costs, and that the study will successfully address a sponsor's goals. By running multiple simple studies as a program rather than as one large study, one can individually control the timing of each component and avoid the scenario where all objectives are placed at risk together.

RANDOMIZED STUDIES DO NOT HAVE TO BE COMPLICATED
With the benefits of treatment with Angiotensin Converting Enzyme (ACE) inhibitors well established for patients with cardiovascular disease, manufacturers of a newer class of agents known as Angiotensin II Receptor Blockers (ARBs) have long recognized the need to validate the non-inferiority of their products versus ACE inhibitors. The difficulty was the need to conduct RCTs with the tens of thousands of patients to ensure statistical significance.

In 2001 Boehringer Ingelheim embarked on this challenge for their ARB product Mycardis (Telmisartan) through the ONTARGET/TRANSCEND program, which consists of two randomized sub-studies both scheduled to report in 2007. By sharing the same research infrastructure and materials between studies, opting for a very simple visit schedule and focusing data collection efforts on major endpoints and safety, this simple research program was able to win significant investigator interest and exceed its recruitment target of 23,400 patients by over 5,000.[2]

Patients in the research program are screened for ACE inhibitor tolerability—those that pass are enrolled into ONTARGET (which includes ACE, placebo, and Mycardis treatment groups), those that fail are enrolled into TRANSCEND (which only involves placebo and Mycardis treatments). Taking this approach has allowed Boehringer to include patients that would otherwise have been ONTARGET screening failures (up to 20 percent of the study population). By conducting two parallel and relatively simple RCT studies, Beohringer is on track to capture the volume of data they need to prove that their product is as effective as the popular ACE inhibitors in treating patients at high risk of heart disease.

Communicate

A study in a vacuum will generate no noise. To achieve maximum value from a study, one must design it to answer the information needs of the market and ensure that its results are communicated to its target audience. Delivery, performance, and timing of strategic research can make or break a commercial strategy. Historically, many pharmaceutical companies have had difficulty clearly managing the coordination of strategic research between clinical and commercial groups, often designing studies with limited value for the market or missing opportunities to maximize communication with the public.

Although clinical research operations are usually charged with designing, executing, and consolidating a study, other stakeholders are also involved in the project. At the beginning, corporate strategists—including representatives from medical affairs, health economics, marketing, sales, and reimbursement—set the key priorities for the product and directions for potential research. At the end, the same group is responsible for maximizing the value of any research conducted. As with any endeavor that involves multiple stages and multiple stakeholders it is important that the study group charge someone with ensuring effective communication and transition of responsibilities between parties.

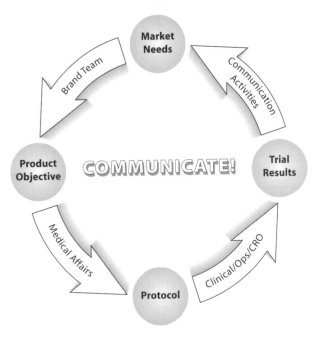

FIGURE 6. The process of Phase IIIB and IV research must be coordinated so that communication activities at the end of the process are ready to start as soon as study results are completed.

Equally important as good internal communication is communication with external stakeholders. The most effective sponsors have members of the brand team create draft publication and communication plans in parallel with their protocols. As each study progresses, they refine these plans with additional detail to maximize public relations opportunities through medical and lay media pickup, and they encourage appropriate use of these results in regulatory negotiations, reimbursement strategies, or the development of marketing plans and materials. A brand team that is isolated from Phase IIIB/IV research planning and execution, and is not prepared to receive study results as they become available, will not be able to work the results effectively into the brand strategy.

Team members must consider a variety of questions. How should results be communicated? Which journals should be targeted for publication? When and how do these journals need to receive manuscripts? How could data be used to maximum effect in continuing medical education programs, newsletters or other sponsored activities? Could sales representatives use interim data to drive field activities? Is corporate public relations involved in the process?

Key opinion leaders play a large role in amplifying research messages. Much time, effort, and money is spent developing them as important leaders for the medical community and press. Some companies actively involve key opinion leaders in their publication planning and communication process, reinforcing the clear messages that were developed during the earlier stages of the research by using these leaders' ability to communicate study results to the media as well as to well-organized seminars and conferences.

GETTING THE RIGHT MESSAGE THROUGH

Publishing a study provides no guarantee that the medical community will notice its results, let alone be satisfied with the objectivity of the research or interpret them in line with a sponsor's expectations. A coordinated communications approach at the time of publication, however, can go a long way to ensuring that good science becomes a good investment. In late 2003, Novartis announced the publication of results from their VALIANT trial—a randomized study of 14,703 patients—that confirmed that its angiotensin II receptor blocker (ARB), Diovan, is as effective as an ACE inhibitor at improving health outcomes when used after a myocardial infarction.[3] The VALIANT study was well timed, positioning DIOVAN as the first ARB to demonstrate therapeutic equivalence with ACE inhibitors and thereby achieving the scientific significance required for publication by the New England Journal of Medicine.

As members of the study's scientific committee, clinical leaders from Harvard and the University of Glasgow provided vocal and public support for the study's results. It clearly bodes well for a product's opportunities when an international scientific leader claims that "even if a newer agent is more expensive, it is welcome news that we now have the option and the alternative, and we should be extending the use to people who are having difficulties with the cheaper, better-used, better-studied, better-known agents."[4]

Conclusion

The key to successful strategic research is understanding what needs to be achieved, then working backwards from this objective toward study design. The objective of registration research is always clear: regulatory approval. Clarifying the objectives of strategic research involves more thought and discipline to balance the needs of different stakeholders. Plan ahead, know your goals, keep the study simple, and make sure you communicate your results in the most effective manner possible. In communicating study results, close attention to the timing of release and the amplification of key messages will help you get the maximum value from your research.

References

1. J&J Press Release, Intravenous administration required when using EPREX/ ERPYO (epoetin alfa) in chronic renal failure patients. Dec 2002, available at http://www.investor.jnj.com/ release Detail.cfm?ReleaseID =96270&year=2002.*

2. Boehringer Ingelheim Press Release: First phase of ONTARGET/TRAN-SCEND cardiovascular protection megatrial completed—All patients enrolled ahead of target. 18 June 2003, available at http://www.ontarget-micardis .com/asp/news/ndetail .asp?ID=874*

3. Novartis Press Release: Leading high blood pressure drug Diovan (valsartan) is also potentially a life-saving treatment after heart attack, major new study finds. 10 Nov 2003, available at http://www.pharma.us.novartis.com/news-room/press Releases/releaseDetail.jsp?PRID=1083; and Pfeffer et al. Valsartan, captopril, or both in myocardial infarction complicated by heart failure, left ventricular dysfunction, or both. N Engl J Med 2003 Nov 13;349(20): 1893–906.

4. Brookes, L. The Valsartan in acute myocardial infarction trial (VALIANT): An expert interview with Marc Pfeffer, MD, PhD, and John JV McMurray, MD. Medscape Cardiology 2003;7(2).

*Note: All citations to websites listed in this book were verified in May of 2005.

7 Minimizing Risk

STRATEGIC RESEARCH IS associated with different risks than registration research. During the course of strategic research, negative data can impact performance of marketed brands, ineffective execution can compromise relationships with the medical profession, and illegal promotion and marketing of approved product can calamitously affect corporate well-being.

Brand Risk

Every study carries a risk of generating negative data that could demonstrate the reverse of what researchers expect. Bristol Myers-Squibb felt the repercussions of a negative outcome in early 2004 when their Prove-It study, comparing Pravachol to Lipitor, showed that their competitor's drug was associated with better health outcomes.[1]

The question, then, is how to counter the risk of negative data. Since all study designs carry a risk of unexpected results, one must balance the risks of proceeding with a particular study against the risks of not proceeding. Clearly, for issues of suspected drug safety, the potential penalties associated with not applying appropriate corporate due diligence could be many times greater than the total sales revenue of a product! On the other hand, the negative market impact of a negative patient preference study might be far greater than any positive impact that positive study results might have generated.

It is important to recognize that the more data is collected, the greater the risk of generating spurious negative analyses. Drug X may perform better than drug Y, but drug X is clearly inferior when used in diabetic patients with amputated toes. Resist the temptation to collect bits and pieces of data that might be interesting: sticking to your key objectives results in simpler, cheaper, and lower risk studies. This is important for reducing the risk of negative data as well as for maximizing the value of the study.

Carefully choose your study design on the basis of what you want the data for, when you want it, and how strong you want any outcomes to be, recognizing that the stronger the study, the more damaging any negative result will be.

Relationship Risk

Conducting research in parallel with commercial activity introduces the possibility of risk to important relationships—including relationships with key opinion leaders, important prescribers, patients, and advocacy groups, and even academic institutions.

Clinical research associates (CRAs) are charged with ensuring protocol compliance, data quality, and appropriate record keeping. As part of this responsibility, CRAs are often required to "encourage" sites to complete their responsibilities, which can often result in increased tension. Most Phase II and III research sites have staff members who are well trained in clinical study processes and understand the role of the CRA in supporting clinical trials. Phase IIIB and IV research frequently involves working with understaffed sites, where staff members often have unrealistic expectations regarding the level of site support that they will need. Working with these research-naive sites means addressing site responsibilities—often directly to the investigator—and requires an additional level of tact and skill on the part of the CRA, who must ensure the integrity of the research project while protecting a valuable investigator relationship.

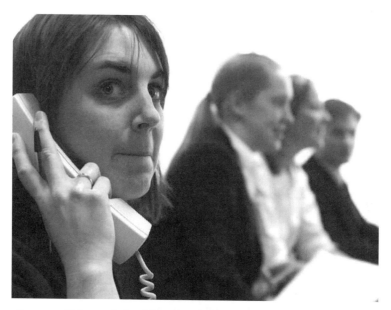

FIGURE 7. Risks to relationships exist whenever there is contact between CRA staff and an investigator's staff. Following up with investigators helps with timely data collection, but care should be taken to respect the busy nature of the primary care environment.

AVOID COMMERCIAL DISASTERS

Many marketers can share their horror experiences with Phase IIIB and IV clinical research activities. Out of the blue, a key opinion leader called to cancel his weekend speaking engagement after a young CRA demanded corrected paperwork. Understandably, the head of marketing, who was left high and dry with no speaker, questioned the value of the study and the competency of the medical affairs team managing the project. In another case, an important prescriber, whose site took five days longer than anticipated to receive a drug, complained to the manufacturer's CEO. Ironically, studies designed to generate strong data and provide reasons to use the product can severely damage relationships if a common sense and mature approach to CRA-level relationship management is not applied.

Negative interactions are easily preventable using well-trained staff and an established protocol for event escalation. CRAs need to be trained to treat investigators in these types of studies with the same courtesy, consideration, and tact that would be used in dealing with important customers, rather than just treating investigators as contractors who need to be pushed to obtain the data for the study. Any complaints from the investigator about his or her treatment during the study need to be escalated quickly to ensure that additional training or site support is provided.

Whether they are dealing with a CRA, a sales representative, or the brand manager, most people view them all as part of one pharmaceutical company and make little distinction between them although their roles are very different. A negative interaction with a CRA, for instance, will reflect poorly on the sponsor as a whole; conflicting messages from CRAs and sales representatives can also reflect poorly on a brand. Market surveys suggest that most CRAs are unaware of the responsibilities of a sales representative and medical science liaison, who frequently call upon the same investigator as they do. The best management of strategic research sites involves open acknowledgement of the different sponsor representatives who make contact with an investigator, and the establishment of communication channels between these individuals.

In designing Phase IIIB and IV studies, it is also important to recognize that onsite CRA time can take away from the amount and quality of time that sites can provide to other sponsor representatives. CRAs, nurse educators, medical science liaisons, and sales representatives are seen as extensions of the same pharmaceutical manufacturer, and many physicians are wary about the amount of time that they spend with each individual company. Studies should be designed to minimize the amount of time that each investigator is required to spend interacting with the CRA and research staff, particularly if the study occurs during a time when sales personnel will be involved in extensive contacts with physicians in the investigator's area of practice. If an investigator feels bombarded by requests for time from a particular company, it can negatively affect their perceptions of that company, its studies, and its products.

Corporate Risk

Phase IIIB and IV research is conducted within a complex regulatory framework, involving a range of regulatory considerations not applicable during Phase II and III. (See chapter 5 and the appendix.) Failure to comply with these laws and regulations can lead to significant civil and criminal penalties. The basic premise behind many of these regulations is that companies must never sponsor or conduct a study that has as one of its aims inducing physicians to prescribe medication.

The Health and Human Services' (HHS) Office of the Inspector General (OIG) has given notification of high risk areas for anti-kickback activity, including consultancy fees, medical education, and clinical research. In 2003, the U.S. Department of Health and Human Services fined TAP Pharmaceuticals $875 million for a range of regulatory violations, including encouraging physicians to bill for medication already supplied by TAP. A number of other companies have since negotiated out-of-court settlements with HHS. Significant financial penalties also exist in other countries for activities that may violate promotional codes or induce inappropriate prescribing.

Key safeguards to minimize corporate risk in Phase IIIB and IV research can be broadly divided into three categories: infrastructure, operations, and leadership.

Infrastructure. Critical to the success of a corporate risk-mitigation strategy is the formal adoption of a core quality standard specific to Phase IIIB and IV research. The standard must address the special needs of research conducted in parallel with commercial activity and must be supplemented with SOPs and formal training activities. The SOPs must include appropriate sensitivity to the different regulatory considerations associated with strategic research and to any relevant geographic variation.

Operations. Highest risk areas for research operations occur at the protocol design stage and at points in the study process where investigators interface with the study—including registration, contracting, materials management, payment, and ongoing support. Building into the operational management of the study both a key risk management checklist and a secondary review process can reduce corporate exposure.

For optimal performance and compliance, someone must see that SOPs are implemented across the board in all studies. Organizations can mistakenly charge a representative from quality assurance with this task; their role, however, should be confined to monitoring compliance, not driving the implementation of SOPs on a project-by-project basis.

Scripting standard interactions between CRAs and investigators (e.g., "when querying slow patient enrollment, open with ... and raise the following three points ...") is a helpful and effective way to minimize miscommunication with sites and maximize regulatory compliance when a large number of CRAs are involved. Scripting could prevent CRAs, who are used to offering incentives to accelerate patient recruitment in registration studies, from doing so in Phase IIIB and IV and risking a violation of the Anti-kickback statute.

Managing good central compliance records, including justification for investigator fees, relevant history, and rationale for commencing the study, is critical to good research practice. It may look suspicious if it takes a company days, rather than hours, to find paperwork in response to a regulator's questions. Research should be separated as much as possible from sales and marketing, and all printed or electronic documents should reflect that separation, particularly in the project design phase.

Leadership. The regulatory environment for strategic research is rapidly changing, affecting all parts of the clinical research process including patient consent, investigator contracting and payment, data collection, and ethics/IRB management. The best way to remain abreast of changes is to engage in the process, using open dialogue and active participation in industry interest groups to see changes on the horizon and respond as necessary.

Conclusion

There are numerous and various risks associated with strategic research that are not considered in the practice of registration research. Sponsors and CROs must consider the risk of negative data in studies that they choose to do; similarly, they must take note of the risk of spoiling relationships with investigators and patients in the process of running the study; and finally they must be attentive to a quickly changing and increasingly constrictive legal environment, including fines and penalties under the Anti-kickback statute that could easily put a drug manufacturer out of business. Understanding the risk areas unique to strategic research is critical to conducting Phase IIIB and IV studies safely.

References

1. Cannon CP, Braunwald E, McCabe CH. The pravastatin or atorvastatin evaluation and infection therapy—Thrombolysis in myocardial infarction 22 investigators: intensive versus moderate lipid lowering with statins after acute coronary syndromes. N Engl J Med 2004.

III Unique Study Dynamics

8 Optimizing Site Performance

THE ENGINE OF MOST clinical trials is the research site. It is here that patients are recruited, their treatments coordinated, and their clinical data captured. Maximizing the efficiency and productivity of research sites, while minimizing the effort required to sustain performance, is the operational aim of most contract research organizations (CROs).

Imagine the research site as a production unit that generates clinical data as a byproduct of patient care. The "production" of data for a particular study represents an extra workload on the normal business of the site. This burden is a function of protocol complexity and operational design—including paperwork load. Depending on the level of research experience and infrastructure available, sites differ in their ability to deal with this workload. The effort required to produce the data is a hurdle that must be overcome through investigator motivation and, possibly, external site support (see figure 8.1).

If investigator motivation is high enough, and sufficient infrastructure is available to overcome this hurdle, sites will perform effectively with very little external support. When this condition is met, studies appear to execute effortlessly.

If, however, investigator motivation or infrastructure are not sufficient, or decrease over time, additional external site support is necessary to pull the site through. Most clinical researchers are

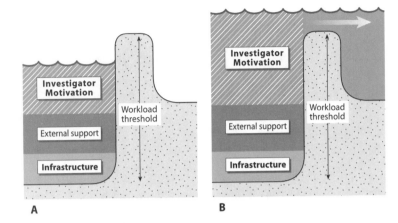

FIGURE 8.1. Drivers of study. For a study to be successful, site infrastructure, investigator motivation, and external support combined must provide enough "energy" to meet the requirements of study workload. Figure A represents a study with insufficient energy; it will not enroll a sufficient number of patients or provide the requisite data.

familiar with studies that require sites to be continually chased for a document or deliverable or where recruitment is always behind target.

Workload and Research Infrastructure

Phase II and III studies usually occur at sites that not only have experience in conducting clinical research but also have an established clinical research infrastructure. These sites, which may do as much "business" conducting research as treating patients, employ study coordinators and research nurses to follow the traditional clinical trials workflow demanded by the pharmaceutical industry.

Sites that have a research infrastructure require less motivation and external support to overcome the hurdle imposed by a study's workload (see figure 8.2). As a result, "simple" study designs seem

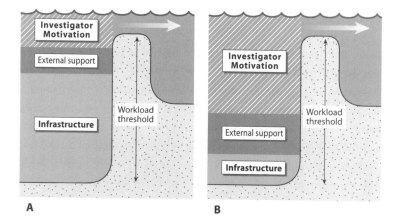

FIGURE 8.2. A research infrastructure provides much of the energy to drive a study (A). The absence of such an infrastructure can be compensated for by increasing investigator motivation and external support (B).

effortless to sites that are well adapted to pharmaceutical research practice and unbelievably burdensome to those that are not.

Sponsors and CROs choose sites for strategic research for reasons that include the number of key opinion leaders at the site, the volume of patients that the site might see, or the site's experience with the disease or medications. Many of these sites will not have research experience or a substantial research infrastructure. Those that do often choose to apply their resources toward the higher paying, earlier phase studies.

Many sponsors are surprised that protocols executed effectively through a small number of well-resourced research sites generate substandard results when opened to a larger group of investigators. It is imperative when planning a study in Phase IIIB and IV that the project workflow be sensitive to the research infrastructure, clinical experience, and clinical practice workflow at each site, and that wherever possible the burden imposed on sites is actively minimized (see chapter 9).

Investigator Motivation

Most investigators who participate in Phase II and III research identify themselves as researchers as well as doctors. These investigators have a natural affinity for research activities and usually need to maintain regular participation in clinical studies to fund quite sizeable research infrastructures. The Phase II and III investigator often actively seeks out studies to participate in, submits study proposals for funding, and is receptive to any new research activity. As a result, site selection strategies for Phase II and III research usually focus on the appropriateness of their infrastructure and patient base, rather than their underlying interest in the study.

As discussed in the previous section, Phase IIIB and IV study designers do not choose sites for strategic research because of the site's commitment to research or supporting infrastructure. Studies designed to translate controlled research findings into a real-world context may actively exclude prominent research sites on the basis that they are not representative of real-world practice. In addition, studies that require large numbers of patients and sites must make use of sites that are not research centers.

Many of the physicians involved in strategic research do not identify themselves as researchers, they participate in research only on an ad hoc basis, and they frequently have little or no research infrastructure to support them. As a result, such investigators are less likely to be motivated to participate in research for the sake of it and require compelling reasons to change their normal work practice to accommodate the burden of a clinical study (see chapter 10).

· · · · ·

External Site Support and Brand Perception

If investigator motivation provides the extra energy needed to meet the study workload, investigators sign up. They complete the forms, they submit data on time, and they stay motivated throughout the study and beyond.

If this condition is not met at the outset or breaks down over time, the study begins to fall apart. It becomes harder and harder to sign investigators up, fewer and fewer investigators get their forms in on time, and CRAs begin to chase the sites to keep bringing in data. Even with this added attention, the quality of the data coming in declines. As investigators start having negative interactions with study staff, the study begins to place relationships at risk.

Sponsors have traditionally responded to an imbalance in the motivation and workload in Phase II and III trials by applying more external support to pull the site along. There are more calls to sites, more newsletters, more graphs highlighting recruitment targets, more monitoring visits, and more contacts to resolve queries. While it is often easier to apply more external resources to these activities than influence investigator motivation or review the study workload, the effect of these largely negative activities on investigator relationships and brand perception can often damage any commercial value that the study would otherwise generate.

Conclusion

In designing strategic research studies, managing the balance between investigator workload, investigator motivation, and site support becomes even more critical to the overall success of a project than in earlier phases of research. Relatively small workloads may still place significant burden on sites without research infrastructure, physicians who do not conduct research as a core business can be harder to motivate on a single-study basis, and investigators may view the process of site contact negatively at a time when companies most want positive brand communication.

By minimizing workload and maximizing motivation, a sponsor can minimize the amount of site support required to pull a site along, resulting in an operational study that presents less risk to critical brand relationships. In chapters 9 and 10, we turn to how these can be practically accomplished.

9   Minimizing Study Workload

EVEN THE SIMPLEST STUDIES can impose a significant workload burden on sites with little research infrastructure. Simplifying the study to reduce workload will reduce the amount of external support and motivation required for sites to perform effectively.

There are 10 principles one can apply to the study preparation process to significantly reduce the workload for sites.

1. Simplify Registration Documents

Having one simple, plain-language registration document reduces paperwork for sites and reduces the number of forms that must be followed up with phone calls. There is no reason why a site contract cannot incorporate confidentiality language or collect tickbox information representing a rudimentary CV that meets the needs of ICH-GCP.

Taking a one-size-fits-all approach to contract negotiation further simplifies this process. Negotiating takes a lot of everyone's time, and is a potential source of conflict with the investigator who may also be an important prescriber. Most companies that have adopted this approach also agree on predetermined add-in language that can be automatically approved on the insistence of an investigator. For example, boilerplate language may need to be added for investigators who are subject to local hospital and pharmacy dispensing fees.

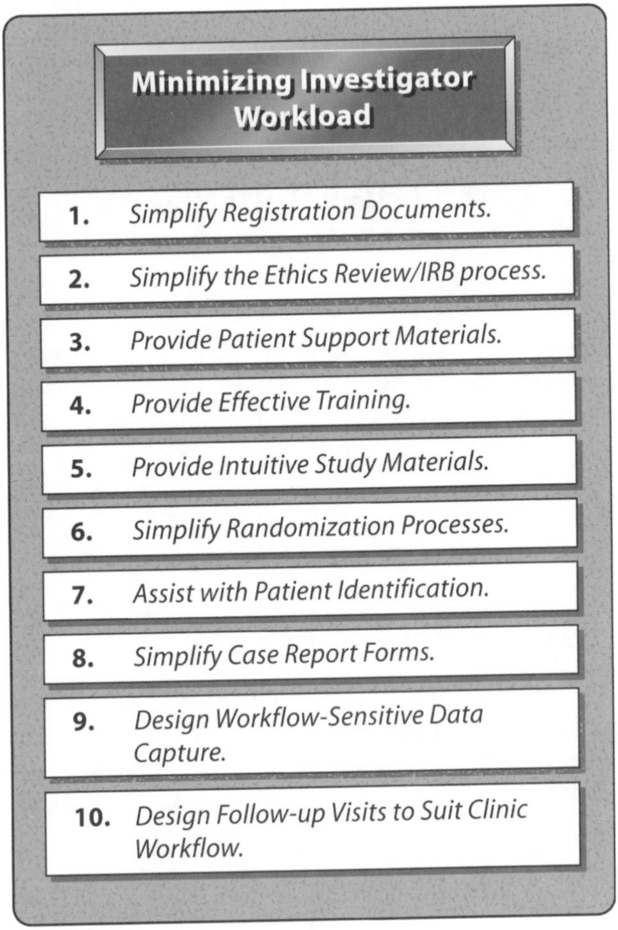

Minimizing Investigator Workload

1. Simplify Registration Documents.

2. Simplify the Ethics Review/IRB process.

3. Provide Patient Support Materials.

4. Provide Effective Training.

5. Provide Intuitive Study Materials.

6. Simplify Randomization Processes.

7. Assist with Patient Identification.

8. Simplify Case Report Forms.

9. Design Workflow-Sensitive Data Capture.

10. Design Follow-up Visits to Suit Clinic Workflow.

FIGURE 9.

2. Simplify the Ethics Review/IRB process

Negotiate a simplified application form with an ethics committee (EC) or independent review board (IRB) that can serve multiple sites. Wherever possible, use this committee and the simplified form, particularly for sites with no EC or IRC structure in place.

Provide a SWAT team that can complete forms and stick "sign here" or "details required" tabs for investigators to complete. For sites that must use the review services of their institution, this SWAT team should obtain a copy of the institution's application form on behalf of the investigator. Even if the investigator must submit the application, the SWAT team should chaperone this process closely and, if required, provide support materials to the investigator in the event that they need to defend their application in front of the review board.

3. Provide Patient Support Materials

Providing sites with materials, such as pamphlets and detail aids, makes it significantly easier for sites to engage patient interest in a study. The materials should describe, in language and a format appropriate for the layperson, the study rationale, schedule of events (including any additional visits or tests), and any patient benefits associated with participation. Many sites note that engaging patient interest and completing the informed consent process place a larger burden on routine clinical practice than any other set of clinical study tasks.

4. Provide Effective Training

It takes much longer to perform a task when you are not sure what you are doing. Sites that do not understand the study workflow, that have not been trained to complete individual study tasks, or that do not understand the key elements of the protocol, take much longer to perform their responsibilities. Even completing a tick-box form requires training and direction. We all know how long it can take to fill in the "simple" immigration forms provided by different countries when we are unfamiliar with them.

When conducting studies that require sites to perform tasks beyond simple data capture, it is critical to provide training for all tasks individually, including tasks such as randomization, physical examination, dispensing medication, and ordering additional study supplies. It is also necessary to train sites in how these tasks relate together within the broader study workflow.

Training can be delivered in a number of different ways. Interactive CD-ROM or internet-based e-learning programs can be effective; however, some objective measure of training completion, such as the submission of a set of test patient forms, is required to ensure that sites have effectively completed the program. Web- and satellite-based meetings can be effective in smaller groups, which can maintain an interactive atmosphere.

Successful training is not just broadcasting information without feedback. Investigator meetings can be valuable for both training purposes and to raise awareness for the science behind the study, but they can be expensive and logistically impossible when working with large numbers of sites. On-site training in parallel with a site screening or activation visit is effective, particularly when a nurse educator rather than a classic CRA delivers the training. Never underestimate the value of an easily accessible help line in providing ongoing support.

Always bear in mind that training is most successful when frequently used and that it is easily forgotten over time; therefore, it is not useful to provide training too far in advance of an anticipated study startup. Keep in mind additional training must also be available to provide for staff turnover, particularly for studies that last longer than six months. If a delay greater than six months is expected between patient enrollments or between patient visits, provision must be made for refresher training. Automated training and testing can help in this situation.

5. Provide Intuitive Study Materials

The more study materials reflect a study workflow, the less training is necessary to ensure protocol compliance. Packaging all study materials together in an attractive and welcoming manner is an important start and reflects a different attitude than traditional black-and-white clinical trial folders with reams of non-carbon duplicate paper and tabbed separators. Simple studies involving single-page registration forms can be more attractively presented as a pad of forms that investigators can fill out and tear off. Patient kits that include CRF (case report form) booklets, diaries, and study medication can help ensure that treatments are appropriately dispensed.

6. Simplify Randomization Processes (or eliminate them)

While randomized controlled designs are still commonly used in Phase IIIB and IV, the process of randomization can frequently be daunting to investigators without research experience. Sites that infrequently participate in clinical research often have difficulty using interactive voice-response telephone randomization systems. They have even more difficulty using internet-based systems. The result is poor protocol compliance and considerable investigator frustration.

If you do not need to use randomization algorithms to tightly balance confounding patient characteristics, you can use strategies that involve randomization by site, with or without crossover, to greatly simplify the workflow for sites and improve protocol compliance. If large patient or site numbers are involved, or if inclusion/exclusion criteria and site selection methods ensure a homogenous study population, you could consider randomizing by site rather than by patient.

7. Assist with Patient Identification

The concept of advertising for patients is not new to clinical research. Increasingly, studies advertise for patients in hospitals and on the radio and television. Sites need to work hard to identify patients when studies have highly selective patient inclusion/exclusion criteria, or involve patients which these sites do not normally see.

One of the most successful strategies in Phase IIIB and IV research is the creation of pseudo-sites. These sites have sufficient knowledge of the study and its selection criteria to identify patients who may be eligible, but they do not collect any data. Patients are not consented but are simply referred to a nearby study site where patient screening and enrollment can take place. As a result, it is not necessary for these sites to go through a formal activation, contract, and ethics/IRB process; they are only subject to confidentiality agreements.

Depending upon the study design, pseudo-investigators may request updates on their patients and ask to receive study newsletters and publications. This approach allows physicians who do not participate in research to offer their patients access to new treatments and tests, and specialist sites can enroll patients for early-intervention studies while maintaining treatment in a primary care setting. The pseudo-investigator approach can help establish referral and communication patterns in support of a product or treatment paradigm (e.g., referral of patients with eczema to centers that offer a specialist treatment).

8. Simplify Case Report Forms

You must develop the simplest case form possible to address the key objectives of the study. Unfortunately, it is much easier to add fields to a form than justify taking them away. Because it is much more expensive, if not impossible, to go back and collect data after the study is completed, all it takes is a suggestion that a particular data point may be useful for it to appear on a case report form. It can take team consensus for it to be removed.

Every data point represents not only another box to be filled in but also work involved in getting the data. Not only do most studies try to capture too much data, but most people involved in these studies will acknowledge that they are trying to capture too much! Taking an indecisive approach toward what data to collect can turn the study into an exercise in detailed but patchy data collection with no prospects for scientifically valid analysis.

Wherever possible, make it easy for investigators to give you clean data. For example, it is easier for an investigator to capture age than birth date. It is easier to collect height and weight than the body mass index. If you are trying to investigate the relationship between a delay in receiving treatment and clinical outcomes, simply ask for how much time elapsed between first onset of symptoms and receipt of treatment. Capturing time and date of both events is a recipe for disaster that creates work for sites and results in very unreliable data.

9. Design Workflow-Sensitive Data Capture

The process of data collection and transfer should not impose a workload burden on investigators. Instead, CROs should attempt to capture data in a workflow sensitive way. Do not ask for test results on a Case Report Form (CRF) when you know that the test referral is only being written that visit. Ask for it on the subsequent visit, or work with a laboratory services provider who will transfer data directly to you. Allow patients to fill out as much of their own data as possible. Provide prepaid envelope or fax services to move data about, but factor in that cheaper model faxes frequently jam after three pages.

I am frequently asked whether or not to use electronic data capture (EDC) for strategic research studies. The answer is simple: not if you expect a doctor to do data entry. Investigators rarely use computers during the consultation process, and expecting a physician to boot up software or go to a specific website during a consultation is difficult to justify. In addition, using such a system requires training and help desk time. This is valuable time taken away from commercial contact opportunities with your sales representatives and medical liaisons.

Between 20 and 50 percent of research-naive sites across the United States and Europe have EDC-compatible information technology infrastructure, but studies involving these sites repeatedly show that only 10 to 20 percent of these sites will actively recruit patients for Phase IIIB and IV research when EDC is the only option provided. When provided with both paper CRFs and an EDC option, as few as 5 percent submit data using EDC. The success of EDC improves dramatically if patients or nurses are available on site to perform data entry. Data from patient diaries and patient-reported outcome forms is consistently well captured by patients using PDAs, tablet PCs, and even cell phones.

10. Design Follow-up Visits to Suit Clinic Workflow

Although patient enrollment may proceed smoothly, follow-up visits impose a significant burden on sites, particularly if many visits are involved over a long period of time. A site needs to develop an effective study-specific filing and patient recall process. A site with 10 patients enrolled in a 12-month study requiring follow-up visits every two months will need to manage 60 recall visits—more than one per week—while getting on with their normal business. As this low-level background work grumbles along, investigator motivation drops rapidly.

Sites need help with their recall responsibilities. For example, sending a weekly fax with a list of all patient IDs scheduled for a recall visit the following week can relieve significant workload. Sending the site forms so that the site does not have to store them—and later dig them up when they are required—can be helpful when a large amount of time elapses between visits. If it is possible to capture data from patient notes, it may be more helpful to send sites batches of follow-up forms every three or six months—one for each patient. Call the site to warn them of an impending batch and follow up days later to ensure completion.

Allowing sites to concentrate their effort in a few, discrete activities a year significantly improves study performance. Sometimes it is not necessary to involve physicians in the follow-up process at all. A study nurse may be provided to run study clinics at a site every month; telephone nurses can call patients to conduct over-the-phone follow-up. One allergy study had physicians remove a postage-paid follow-up postcard from the baseline CRF and give it to patients to complete after seven days to report any adverse symptoms experienced with treatment. Every baseline CRF and postcard was paired and numbered. Ironically, the patients did a better job than the physicians in returning their data. The CRO received thirty percent more patient-completed postcards than physician-completed baseline CRFs.

Conclusion

Phase IIIB and IV studies do not benefit from the same level of investigator motivation and site resources as Phase II and III research, and, therefore, their success is very sensitive to investigator workload. Do your best to minimize workload: simplify forms and processes; provide appropriate training and support materials; and plan study workload to suit the Phase IIIB/IV clinical setting.

Different investigators "feel" the same workload differently depending upon their research experience, specialty, persona, and facility. Before making a substantial investment in study materials and investigator recruitment, perform a small feasibility study involving 10 to 20 sites to ensure that workload is well balanced by other compensating factors.

10 Maximizing Investigator Motivation

INVESTIGATOR MOTIVATION IS A critical factor in the operational success of a clinical study. While many factors that influence investigator motivation are outside the scope of study design or implementation—such as an investigator's natural interest in research or the number of other competing research studies in the same therapeutic area—there are a handful of key study attributes that measurably and significantly drive investigator interest.

The attributes of a study that contribute to investigator motivation, from most to least important, are (1) the benefit to the patient, (2) scientific immediacy, and (3) financial compensation. Optimizing these attributes to maximize investigator motivation can be a simple and efficient way to save on external site support costs, and can result in a self-driving study with a momentum that allows for increased design complexity.

Benefit to the Patient

The greatest driver by far of investigator motivation is the benefit that accrues to patients who participate in a study. Whatever their level of research experience, investigators are physicians concerned primarily with the improvement of patient care. All studies involve some level of inconvenience for a patient, even if this is only additional data collection. Many studies involve multiple

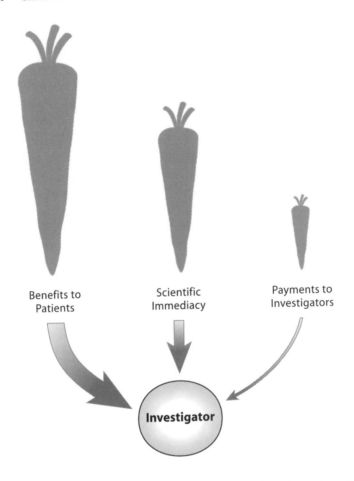

FIGURE 10.1: Investigators tend to be motivated to perform the study work-load if the study provides new benefits to their patients or if it is scientific-ally relevant to their practice. Financial compensation has the smallest effect on motivating investigators to start and complete a study.

additional visits to a clinic and additional tests, some painful. Not many patients like being guinea pigs for the sake of it. It is much easier, and more pleasant, to offer study participation to a patient as a chance to obtain a benefit, rather than in the context of a patient's duty to science and research. If insurance or government programs are not yet paying for drugs or procedures, providing them free of charge can be a very strong driver of patient recruitment.

Patient benefits usually take the form of one or more of the following:

- Access to treatment that is not yet approved
- Access to treatment that is not reimbursed
- Access to tests that are not widely available
- Access to tests that are not reimbursed
- Access to services that are not reimbursed
- Financial compensation

Investigators are highly motivated to participate in Phase II and III studies, which offer patients access to treatments not yet approved by regulators. Many investigators, particularly in oncology, rheumatology, and infectious diseases, participate in earlier phase research to offer patients access to experimental treatments. It has become increasingly difficult for sponsors to recruit patients for studies on experimental treatments not clinically or pharmacologically different from other products already available.

Those planning strategic research activities in Phases IIIB and IV should be mindful of designing studies to maximize patient benefit. A pre-approval Phase IIIB program has a good chance of strong enrollment by offering product that is not yet available. Once approval is obtained, expect that investigator and patient motivation will rapidly diminish. If the workload of the study is not designed to taper off in line with market approval, study managers will need to use a significant amount of external support at the tail end of a study to compensate. The same principle applies for studies started immediately after marketing approval but before reimbursement. External factors can rapidly change the relative benefit of a study to patients, and thus can indirectly but significantly influence investigator motivation and study performance.

Scientific Immediacy

Of next greatest importance to investigator motivation is the scientific immediacy of the study. The investigator will benefit from knowing how relevant and timely the study's scientific questions are to his or her day-to-day practice. Investing a little time to produce site-recruitment materials, protocol synopses, and protocol introductions that highlight the clinical value of the study will pay off many times over in the course of the project.

Scientific immediacy should not be confused with absolute scientific importance. For example, a regulator or sponsor may be keen to demonstrate the safety of a cholesterol-lowering drug in pregnancy—a valid question of broad scientific importance. Because general practitioners do not prescribe cholesterol-lowering medication to pregnant women on a daily basis, however, the immediate application of this research to their practice may not seem significant. On the other hand, obstetricians who specialize in the management of diabetic patients with high cholesterol may recognize a far greater scientific immediacy of the study.

Scientific immediacy also implies a timeliness of analysis. A five-year study, without an interim analysis, is far less motivating than a one-year study with regular interim analysis and communication of results, even if the research objective of the one-year study has much less clinical significance.

Scientific immediacy, like patient benefit, is an important attribute that can be affected by external factors over time. In designing long studies, one should recognize that scientific immediacy decreases over time. Design the study so that patient benefit, financial incentives, or external support increase, or study workload decreases, to compensate for this change.

Sponsors frequently ask me whether they can use sales force or medical liaisons to perform some of the clinical workload. My response is simple. Even ignoring the possible legal and regulatory dangers of having sales representatives participate in studies, the talents of a sales representative are better used elsewhere. Sales representatives and medical liaisons can be more effective in facilitating clinical operations by enhancing the scientific immediacy of a study rather than by helping with the study process itself.

For example, recruitment for a study is significantly enhanced if the media has recently highlighted a related healthcare or clinical issue. Physicians are more likely to recruit patients into a study investigating the relationship between dose at the onset of aura and severity of migraine if sales representatives present data suggesting that many patients with crippling migraine do not receive maximum doses of therapy. Similarly, a medical education campaign focused on increased cardiovascular risk in association with high cholesterol will measurably improve site participation in a study investigating the safety of a lipid-lowering treatment.

Most sponsors will be running a range of educational and communication activities in parallel with their Phase IIIB and IV research. Using these activities to highlight a health issue being tackled by a parallel research study will create significant synergy between the two programs without requiring a direct linkage.

Financial Reward

Surprisingly, for many investigators, payment is not a powerful driver of motivation. Investigators find it hard to enroll patients on the basis that their participation will be lucrative for the site.

Although it is often easier to offer more money, it may be more effective to change the research direction of the study, simplify it, or add features that may increase the benefit for patients.

Quite recently, a sponsor started a large observational study for a marketed product. The sponsor did not provide the investigational drug, reasoning that it was available through commercial channels, but investigators were paid approximately $100 per visit to complete monthly safety review forms. This study had difficulty recruiting from day one because it had limited scientific immediacy and no short-term patient benefit. After recognizing these problems, the sponsor began to provide study drug through a pharmacy coupon program (valued at approximately $100 a month) and eliminated investigator payments to remain budget neutral. Even though investigators no longer received payment, patient recruitment accelerated so significantly that the study completed ahead of schedule.

While some payment is usually necessary to cover the fixed site costs associated with a study, it is my experience that spending an additional $100 on site payments is less motivating than offering $20 of additional value to the patient. I have been involved in many successful studies that required little external support and no payment to investigators at all. They enrolled between 10,000 and 60,000 patients on the basis of strong patient benefit and interesting science.

· · · · ·

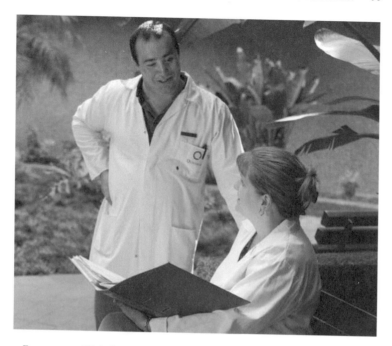

FIGURE 10.2 Clinical researchers. An essential part of running a trial successfully is motivating investigators.

Conclusion

It is my strong recommendation that teams design studies to minimize workload, maximize patient benefit, and promote scientific
immediacy before performing a basic feasibility study to determine the investigator-fee structure necessary to achieve the
desired site behavior. Not only will this approach save significant
amounts of money for the sponsor, but in regions where increased
scrutiny is applied to research payments made in parallel with
commercial activity, a lower, well-documented, and justified fee
structure could protect against enormous penalties (see the
appendix).

11 Working with Market Changes

CHAPTERS 9 AND 10 presented practical guidelines on how to design an effective study. This chapter will further explore how market changes can impact studies, and discuss strategies to recognize and address these changes.

Great differences separate the pre- and post-approval research environments. The pre-approval research environment is relatively static. The study drug is not registered and is not the subject of parallel commercial communications. The drug generally represents a new therapeutic opportunity removed from the competitive "in market" world. Although other experimental compounds may occasionally compete for patient enrollment in studies, such competition is often temporal rather than commercially aggressive.

Things begin to change after a company files for market authorization. Commercial engines start to wind up and indirectly begin to introduce the drug to the market. Product approval is around the corner, and the perceived benefit of accessing the latest drug has started to wear off. Reimbursement is usually not far away. In parallel, competitors are talking up their own drugs and talking down the new market entrant. After market authorization is granted, things change further as the relative calm surrounding a study drug in Phase III gives way to the noise of a competitive commercial battlefield.

Changing Patient Benefit

Since Phase IIIB and IV studies are so sensitive to investigator motivation, any changes in an investigator's perception of patient benefit or scientific immediacy are liable to rapidly affect study performance. Recruitment for a Phase IIIB study will drop rapidly after receipt of marketing approval. Recruitment for a Phase IV study that offers study drug will drop rapidly after reimbursement has been obtained. In addition, safety concerns raised in the market about a competitor can positively or negatively impact patient recruitment and follow-up performance.

Dynamically managing study drivers in a complex market environment is critical to the success of a study. This is the role of a Phase IIIB or IV project manager.

Changing Scientific Immediacy

While the market might have a great scientific interest in a subject today, it is likely that interest will wane quickly. For example, confronted with a slew of new products for the treatment of bipolar depression, the medical community might be crying out for optimal dose management information. Six to twelve months later, after physicians have developed experience with their favorite product or a competitor has released definitive data, the collective sense of interest in the subject will decrease and site performance for a bipolar depression dosing study will begin to flag.

The more data that can be analyzed and presented to investigators, the greater the chance of prolonging scientific interest in the study. Building shorter sub-studies into the main study can provide a sense of pace and energy throughout the project. Building in secondary objectives and additional data points can support interesting interim analyses and generate communication opportunities in the form of newsletters, publications, and even field-force activity.

Communicating results can improve scientific immediacy. Interim analyses, publications, media activity, conferences, and educational events can make the study more significant to the physicians who are collecting data. Adding new scientific dimensions to a study can also revive interest even if it involves a little more work for investigators.

Managing Long Studies

The longer the duration of a study, the more likely that patient benefit and scientific immediacy will diminish as a result of market activity. Recognizing that investigator motivation will naturally decline, one compensates in one of three ways.

1. Diminish workload over time.

This is by far the simplest approach that delivers the best results. The randomized control study can switch to an open-label naturalistic follow-up study after one year. The naturalistic study requires minimal data collection, and the number of CRF pages for patient visits can be reduced to one or two pages.

2. Revive the study with additional motivators.

This tends to be the most effective approach when trying to rescue stalled studies, those in which ongoing patient recruitment or site performance have taken a sudden dive.

If you can add a patient benefit without adding bias to the study, do so, for it can quickly revitalize recruitment. Build in an additional test that the patient may value; incorporate a nurse/health counselor so patients get more face time with a health professional. Even add a little patient support kit to the process (consisting of a video, pens, and reading material about the disease).

3. Pay investigators more.

As a method of last resort, site payments can be increased to compensate for diminishing investigator motivation and decreasing scientific immediacy that creeps in over the course of a project. If it is necessary to increase site payments to collect the necessary data, the reasons for the increase must be well documented and the increase itself must be consistent among all sites.

Window on the World

Strategic studies represent an excellent barometer of clinical sentiment because they are so sensitive to market changes. In the weeks immediately following the Vioxx recall, Novartis or Pfizer could have used recruitment rates in their larger IIIB and IV studies to examine whether the market was switching to other COX-IIs or away from them completely.

This linkage between strategic studies and the market can even be used to make regulatory arguments. One top-five pharmaceutical company successfully used diminishing study recruitment rates to convince regulators that physicians and patients were no longer concerned about a particular safety issue for their product.

IV Special Cases of Strategic Research

12 Registries

OFTEN DESCRIBED AS "looking over a doctor's shoulder," a registry technically speaking is a prospective open-label observational study. A registry includes a naturalistic record of patient characteristics, treatment decisions, and clinical outcomes that can be used to identify important trends through a variety of data mining techniques. Registries are passive non-experimental data collection exercises that do not influence or dictate treatment decisions. They are a special type of an observational study that does not require particular investigations or a strict follow-up schedule since the very process of doing so might influence clinical behavior.

Registries broadly fall into the following three categories, each of which has different research objectives: product registries, disease registries, and exposure registries. Even though they are not retrospective studies themselves, registries frequently involve collection of retrospective data at baseline, like product use history, disease history, or exposure history, before the collection of prospective data begins.

Types of Registries

Product Registries

In general, product registries lead to data that can be used to generate product guidelines. Product registries enroll patients receiving a particular treatment, and they often restrict participation to patients with certain demographic and medical characteristics. Product registries commonly address questions relating to the "best practice" use of a product, and are generally conducted when market uptake is limited by lack of knowledge or confidence in the product. For example, market adoption of a new, more potent protease inhibitor for the treatment of HIV may be delayed if physicians do not feel comfortable switching patients from an older drug to the new agent.

Product registries can be used to help define patient characteristics that positively and negatively predict for treatment success with a particular product. They can also assist in defining treatment expectations and health outcomes for prescribers and patients, establishing product dosing and optimal duration of treatment, identifying additional properties of a drug, and monitoring a product's safety profile in a broader population as part of a risk management plan.

Evaluating Safety in Pregnancy

Conducting clinical trials with pregnant or breastfeeding women is usually considered unethical, but characterizing the relative safety of drugs in pregnancy remains very important. This is particularly true for drugs that cannot be justifiably discontinued even for short periods of time, such as treatments for epilepsy, schizophrenia, cardiac arrhythmias, and asthma. Registries remain the most common way that manufacturers can assess the safety of their products in pregnancy. Sponsors invite doctors to enroll pregnant patients who are receiving treatment despite the relative contraindication of pregnancy. GlaxoSmithKline (GSK) initiated its International Lamotrigine Pregnancy Registry in 1992 to monitor pregnancies exposed to lamotrigine (LTG), an anti-epileptic, for the occurrence of major birth defects. By March 2004, GSK was able to analyze data from 414 patients exposed to lamotrigine monotherapy during their first trimester and demonstrate that the risk of all major birth defects was similar to that in the general population.[1]

Disease Registries

Disease registries generate data that can be used to better establish disease treatment guidelines. Disease registries involve enrollment of patients who have been diagnosed with a particular disease, often restricting participation to patients with certain demographic and clinical characteristics. Disease registries are commonly performed when the market is unsure of a treatment's place in the management of a disease. When should patients undergoing knee surgery be offered treatment with a new anticoagulant approved for the prevention of deep venous thrombosis in an orthopedic setting? At what age does the benefit of treating patients with high cholesterol outweigh the risks? Should product X be used first or second line, and what are the criteria for diagnosing first-line treatment failure?

Investigators often initiate disease registries, sometimes as informal programs conducted at individual practices. Such registries are common in fast-evolving therapeutic areas, such as oncology, neurology, and rheumatology, where there is no gold standard treatment. Disease registries also target diseases associated with large variations in clinical outcomes or very small patient numbers, such as HIV, cystic fibrosis, and Tay-Sachs disease.

Disease registries can be powerful in establishing or defining new disease states that were previously unrecognized as coincidental collections of unrelated symptoms or different variants of normal. Such registries enroll patients exhibiting a particular set of clinical characteristics, and they track progress over time to see if there is

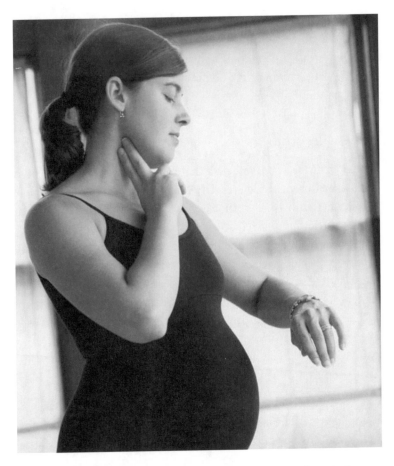

FIGURE 12. Registries, which simply observe the outcomes of standard care, are often the only ethical way to evaluate the safety of medicines in pregnancy.

a collective association with unfavorable patient outcomes over the long term. Short concentration span and behavioral difficulties in children may not be considered medical problems in themselves, but demonstrating an association between these characteristics and long-term patient outcomes that clearly fall outside the normal range can establish this constellation of symptoms as a disease with a rationale for treatment.

IMPROVING TRANSPLANT OUTCOMES

The International Pancreas Transplant Registry (IPTR), supported by grants from the National Institutes of Health and Roche, is one of the longest running registries. Established in 1980, the registry has worked closely with pancreatic transplant institutions around the world to record almost all pancreatic transplants performed since the first in 1969. The registry now has records of over 24,000 patients. The IPTR has been influential in better understanding the changing approaches to surgical treatment of diabetes mellitus and in identifying best practices to improve treatment outcomes and patient survival. Data from the IPTR has supported the development of simultaneous pancreas and kidney transplants, improvements in the management of immunosuppression, and identification of donor and recipient risk factors for treatment failure.[2]

Exposure Registries

Exposure registries lead to data that can be used to prove association (but not causality) between an exposure and a health outcome. Exposure registries enroll patients who have been exposed to a particular product, place, or thing, and attempt to capture data over time to demonstrate association between exposure and risk of different clinical outcomes.

Investigators commonly perform exposure registries when trying to understand the etiology of a particular disease, and epidemiologists frequently use them to identify any particular characteristics of an exposure that modify patient risk. Are Gulf War veterans or World Trade Center survivors at increased risk for developing particular diseases? If so, what characteristics of their exposure place them at increased risk? Do children of mothers who took a particular product prior to or during pregnancy have an increased risk of developing certain pathologies? Is the measles, mumps, and rubella vaccine related to an increased risk of autism?

SEPTEMBER 11TH REGISTRY

Following the September 11th attack on the World Trade Center (WTC), many New Yorkers were naturally concerned about the long-term effects of the disaster on their physical and mental well-being. The WTC Registry enrolled over 71,000 people who were either located near the site at the time of the disaster or involved in rescue or clean-up activities in the aftermath. Consisting of a telephone interview and periodical follow-up calls, the registry is designed to track and investigate possible trends in illness and recovery, and to help create guidelines that can save lives and reduce injuries in future disaster settings.[3]

Exposure registries frequently mix retrospective and prospective components. The registries collect a large amount of retrospective data at baseline about the exposure (which frequently has occurred months or years in the past). Some exposure registries collect follow-up data over time to determine if a temporal relationship exists between exposure and a given health outcome—as was found to be the case with asbestos exposure and mesothelioma.

Analytical Opportunities

By passively collecting data, often over long periods of time, registries can produce excellent data sets to support quantitative and descriptive analyses that aim to identify hypothetical trends. Registries can often generate strong empirical evidence of association through retrospective case-control analyses and are routinely used to influence product-safety label changes. Registries frequently lead to excellent and ongoing publication opportunities in scientific journals. Beginning with a cross-sectional analysis of baseline data, analytic teams can support a range of communication activities across the lifecycle of the research project.

Investigator Dynamics

How can you motivate investigators to do registry work? By definition, registries do not influence treatment, investigations, or follow-up. As a result, it is impossible to provide free drug, free tests, or additional services as part of a registry, diminishing any potential patient benefit associated with participation in the study. Registries frequently require many thousands of patients in order to produce a large enough data set for analysis. This limits the amount of payment that can realistically be made to physicians for data collection.

With patient benefits and financial rewards diminished as possible investigator motivators, study designers need to rely on scientific immediacy to compensate for study workload. Reducing this study workload to the extreme is a critical part of the registry design process as well. Even simple registries can experience slow patient enrollment because workload still places too much burden on sites.

Scientific immediacy can be maximized by clearly establishing the objectives of a registry in a market relevant context, providing examples of questions that the registry hopes to address, and committing to a timeline for communication of results. Obviously, this immediacy is further increased through a strategic selection of investigators most interested in the scientific objectives of the study.

Investigators can limit the burden to sites by streamlining site registration activities through simplified documentation and centralized ethics/IRB approval. Other approaches include supporting the process of patient consent by providing enrollment brochures that describe the scientific value of the study, and applying work-flow sensitive follow-up designs that may involve creative methods of data collection. It is sometimes possible for an ethics committee to waive the need for informed patient consent when the registry has no impact on medical treatment. By wrapping a registry in appropriate medical and lay public relations activity, which focuses on the market relevant questions that the study intends to answer, one can both increase the scientific immediacy of the study and generate positive attention in support of a brand.

Pitfalls

Registries have gained popularity within the industry as a generic, commercially attractive Phase IV study because they are associated with small payments to investigators and no requirement to provide study drug. Some companies calculate their return on investment from a registry on the basis of "number of patients times number of scripts," in possible violation of the Anti-kick-back statute (see the appendix) and completely miss the enormous value that market relevant research findings may have on product sales. Other companies can damage sales force relationships by assigning negatively perceived administrative tasks, such as collecting forms, to sales representatives as an excuse for increased clinical contact. It would be better to provide them with tools to facilitate communication of study results back to investigators.

Many companies conduct "catch all" registries that have no clear research goals and market-relevant objectives. Sometimes an armful of objectives are lumped together to avoid the cost of conducting multiple studies. These registries rarely generate useful scientific data.

A registry that lacks scientific immediacy is often marked by a good start followed by poor ongoing performance. Before the launch of the study, internal brand team excitement fuels expectations. Site enrollment proceeds to plan, but within the first 8 to 12 weeks it becomes clear that patient recruitment is not making the expected numbers. Repeated contact with sites to increase patient enrollment begins to strain investigator relationships, and the sales team begins to receive negative feedback. Confronted with this situation, companies attempt to recover by increasing investigator fees without considering the key drivers of investigator motivation: patient benefit and scientific immediacy. Instead of focusing on these motivators, companies significantly increase study costs without dramatically improving site performance. In contrast, academically driven registries with well-established, market relevant scientific objectives can easily attract 50,000 plus patients without offering any payment, by applying these key principles too often forgotten in industry registries.

Regulatory Issues

Since registries are vehicles for passive data collection that have no influence on patient care, ethical issues associated with registries are normally limited to the data collection process and relevant privacy considerations. Many countries do not require ethics approval for registries; those that do typically use the process to ensure that the study is limited to passive data collection only.

Because the conduct of a registry does not place patient safety at risk, monitoring to ensure protocol compliance is unnecessary. Monitoring is only necessary to ensure data quality and completeness, and to protect against malicious activity. Infrequent monitoring is the rule, and "for cause" on-site visits are reserved for cases of suspected fraud. In many registries, particularly disease and exposure registries, the only monitoring done is remote "for cause" monitoring, initiated when outlying data points need confirmation to ensure accuracy.

References

1. Cunnington, Marianne, Tennis, Patricia, and the International Lamotrigine Pregnancy Registry Scientific Advisory Committee. Lamotrigine and the risk of malformations in pregnancy. Neurology. Mar 2005;64:955–960.

2. http://www.iptr.umn.edu/IPTR/home.html.*

3. http://www.wtcregistry.org.*

Note: All citations to websites listed in this book were verified in May of 2005.

13   Expanded Access Programs

EXPANDED ACCESS PROGRAMS, also known as "early access" or "compassionate use" programs, provide access to unapproved products for patients with life threatening or significant illnesses. They usually take place during Phase IIIB after a general safety profile for the product has been established. Expanded access programs do not have a research rationale, but can provide an opportunity for a large scale assessment of risk/benefit for products that have not been fully evaluated by regulators.

For the community, expanded access programs provide patients with months, and sometimes years, of access to life-improving or life-saving treatments. In addition to their public benefit, expanded access programs offer pharmaceutical companies an opportunity to provide prescribers with pre-market product experience. Companies can establish a base of patients who will already be on treatment once approval has been granted, and sometimes they can collect additional safety data that may be used to supplement the original NDA submission.

The regulatory framework for expanded access programs varies dramatically between countries; this is true even within Europe, where the European Medicines Evaluation Agency (EMEA) has attempted to harmonize approaches to pharmaceutical regulation. Expanded access programs can take one of three approaches: the clinical trial approach, the named patient approach, and the cohort approach.

<small>IMPROVING ACCESS TO TREATMENT</small>
In March 2002, as Gilead Sciences was preparing to submit marketing authorization applications for adefovir dipivoxil (Hepsera) to treat chronic Hepatitis B, the company also announced the initiation of an expanded access program. The program was designed to provide Hepsera as a therapeutic alternative for patients with lamivudine-resistant chronic Hepatitis B infection not suitable for treatment with interferon-alpha. Gilead made Hepsera available to patients 16 years or older with chronic Hepatitis B infection resistant to lamivudine and who were at risk for disease progression. Participation was subject to evaluation at baseline, after one month on therapy, and every two months thereafter. The Hepsera expanded access program continued until the drug obtained marketing approval in the United States (September 2002) and Europe (March 2003), by which time over 1600 patients had been enrolled in the program.[1]

Clinical Trial Approach

The clinical trial approach establishes a prospective observational protocol with one treatment arm for the expanded access product. There are no endpoints and no limits to sample size. In most markets, this approach requires that the program be executed in the same way as a normal clinical study. In the United States, sponsors must proceed by submitting a special investigational new drug application known as a treatment IND. The program protocol is usually filed under the treatment IND, which is granted on the basis of medical need.

An expanded access program using the clinical trial approach requires approval by ethics committees in the usual manner. The ethics committee will review the risk/benefit posed by the protocol rather than the usual research rationale. Data collection is usually limited to the collection of safety information. The protocol must define strict inclusion/exclusion criteria for participation in the program, as well as mandate any necessary patient monitoring required to maximize safety. Study monitoring is almost always confined to monitoring of inclusion/exclusion criteria to ensure that the product is used in a manner approved by the ethics committee.

The clinical trial approach places responsibility for tracking adverse events with the program sponsor, creating a dual-edged sword. On the one hand, sponsors remain in control of this pharmacovigilance data and can manage their product safety strategies accordingly; on the other hand, they are bound by the same adverse event reporting and medico-legal obligations as for other clinical trials. A higher than expected rate of serious adverse events, which can occur because the expanded access protocol is less controlled than a standard clinical trial, can jeopardize the breadth of a product label. In addition, holding a large amount of adverse event data on file can increase a company's medico-legal risk in the future.

Named Patient Approaches

Named patient approaches represent a regulatory compromise that allows physicians to seek regulatory approval for patient treatment on a case-by-case basis. Named patient approaches are commonly used in Europe, although the mechanics of each approach still varies from country to country. In the United States, the Emergency Use IND allows physicians to seek case-by-case treatment approval, although the FDA discourages this approach for large programs. In Australia, the Therapeutic Goods Administration provides named patient access through the Special Access Scheme (SAS). In most cases, manufacturers can streamline the named patient process for physicians by centralizing administrative resources and supporting the submission of individual patient applications on behalf of the physician.

The named patient approach toward expanded access requires less setup effort than the clinical trial approach. There is usually no protocol involved, and ethics committee approval is often not required although I have seen a growing expectation from regulators that physicians document risk management plans as part of the application process. Importantly, named patient approaches place greater responsibility for appropriate patient care on the medical community. Adverse event reporting usually follows the same approach as spontaneous post-marketing reporting, with investigators notifying the regulatory agency directly. While this can significantly diminish workload for a sponsor, there exists a disadvantage that the regulator has access to safety data that the sponsor does not.

Cohort Approach

The cohort approach is the simplest way of conducting an expanded access program, but it is currently limited to only a handful of countries such as France and Italy. Regulatory agencies require a special application from a sponsor, but they do not demand that physicians apply on behalf of individual patients. In effect, the cohort approach is tantamount to highly restricted regulatory approval, with significant responsibility resting with the physician to evaluate the appropriateness of treatment on the basis of available data and on an individual patient's condition. In

France, companies can apply for a cohort ATU (Autorisations Temporaires d'Utilisation or Temporary Authorization for Use) at the time that they submit their application for marketing authorization. The cohort ATU allows companies to make their products available for restricted use, while committing them to a program of regular progress reporting and pharmacovigilance activity for the duration of the program.

Reimbursement

Most markets provide manufacturers with the ability to recover costs from patients or insurance companies for products provided within an expanded access program. The cohort ATU in France allows companies to seek full reimbursement from the government pharmaceutical benefits scheme. In the United States, where insurers are reluctant to add non-approved products to their formularies, some companies have chosen to recover costs directly from patients. Although a sponsor can recoup some of the costs associated with running expanded access programs, pre-approval prices have historically been significantly lower than post-approval prices obtained for similar treatments, and there is little opportunity to renegotiate higher prices after approval has been granted.

Investigator Dynamics

Expanded access programs do not offer scientific immediacy or financial payment, but they do offer a significant patient benefit—the opportunity to access a treatment that is not yet publicly available. Since most programs address patients with life-threatening or debilitating diseases for which limited treatment opportunities exist, patients' motivation to participate is extraordinarily high. Irrespective of the workload imposed on investigators, site motivation is also high and over-subscription is common. Over-motivation of sites can result in significant investigator disappointment when program entry is capped or subsidy discontinued. Over-motivation of sites can present deeper problems than under-motivation of sites because it can result in a negative attitude toward a sponsor's whole product line as opposed to impacting only study performance.

Pitfalls

Providing subsidized product represents a significant cost to a sponsor. Running a program for a product that costs only $100 per month, in anticipation of marketing approval twelve months later, is an investment of $1,200 per patient in product alone. For every 1,000 patients enrolled in the expanded access program, the sponsor must make a $1.2 million commitment. A year delay in approval can cost the sponsor the same amount again.

High drug costs drive most pharmaceutical companies to limit enrollment by region, type of physician, and number of patients per site. Because of the over-motivation normally associated with these programs, managing investigator expectations regarding caps and quotas is a difficult and sensitive process. How do you tell a key opinion leader keen to offer more patients access to the life-saving properties of a new drug that their cap has been reached? How do they communicate this to their patients?

A delay in market approval can place a sponsor in a difficult position. It is not uncommon for delays of six to twelve months to cost between $1,000 and $5,000 per patient. Multiply this by 5,000 to 10,000 patients enrolled in a successful program, and a market delay can cost up to $50 million in additional drug alone. The alternate is canceling access to a truly life-improving drug, resulting in such bad feelings from patients and physicians toward a manufacturer that sales of their other brands may be affected.

PUBLIC RELATIONS AND EXPANDED ACCESS

Managing public expectations regarding the limitations of expanded access activities can be a difficult commercial exercise. In 1997 Glaxo Wellcome announced the initiation of a 2,500-patient expanded access program for Abacavir, a promising new antiviral agent for the treatment of HIV. With only a limited range of HIV treatments available at the time, and with over 30,000 patients in the United States alone likely to qualify for treatment, patient activists severely criticized Glaxo for the size of the program. In June 1997 the AIDS activist group ACT-UP seized the investor relations office of Glaxo Wellcome in New York, leading to numerous arrests. In parallel the group coordinated a boycott of Glaxo products including Zantac and Zovirax through a mass-mailing campaign to doctors and politicians. The group called off the boycott after Glaxo executives agreed to meet with advocacy leaders to discuss changes to the program.

Confronted with a possible catastrophic loss of goodwill, sponsors frequently choose to keep programs going in the face of authorization delays. Any pharmaceutical company considering an expanded access program must factor in a delay of between six and twelve months for approval and have a clear, up-front commitment to physicians regarding the size and length of the program in the absence of marketing approval. If it is necessary to end the program, a step-down approach is more palatable than sudden cancellation. Do this initially by limiting resupply to patients already enrolled.

It is good practice to involve a set of key opinion leaders in a steering committee from the beginning. The steering committee should participate in the design of the program and should be aware of total budget and cost of supply, so that they can take responsibility for establishing quotas. Having an independent steering committee can cushion negative market sentiment when expanded access programs need to be limited or delays in regulatory approval forces sponsors to reevaluate program costs.

References

1. Gilead Sciences press release, "Hepatitis B Drug Hepsera™ Approved for marketing in European Union," March 11, 2003, available at http://www.gilead.com/wt/sec/pr_1047342957.*

2. Grinberg L, James JS. 1592 access: larger program planned. AIDS Treat News 1997 Nov 21;(283): 2–3.

Note: All citations to websites listed in this book were verified in May of 2005.

14 Post-Marketing Surveillance

PRE-APPROVAL REGISTRATION TRIALS are usually randomized controlled trials conducted in highly selected patient populations. The limited size and diversity of the population being studied and the short duration of therapy limits the ability of these studies to characterize a drug's safety profile. As an extreme example, imagine a three-month randomized study of smoking for the short-term treatment of obesity in young men and women with no respiratory medical history. Such a study could demonstrate a statistically significant weight-loss effect without revealing the sinister safety profile of cigarette smoking.

When granting approval to new products, regulators—and ultimately prescribers—must make the assumption that pre-registration studies have the potential to elicit safety signals likely to be present with real-world. Of course, the assumption that pre-registration data adequately characterizes a product's long-term real-world safety profile is not wholly accurate. Drug approval represents a balance between protecting public safety and making new products available for patients to use.

Unlike registration trials, which are limited in their ability to track product usage for long periods of time or in diverse populations, post-marketing surveillance (PMS) activities are designed to monitor the safety of products used in the uncontrolled, real-world, post-approval environment. They are meant to ensure that the drug's safety profile does not significantly differ from that

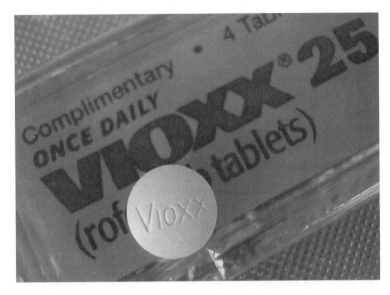

FIGURE 14. Following the withdrawal of Vioxx, post-marketing surveillance programs are receiving renewed attention as companies attempt to demonstrate their best efforts at corporate due diligence.

upon which marketing approval was granted. In some cases surveillance has led to product withdrawals, for example Vioxx, Baycol, and Fen-Phen, and in others it has resulted in significant restriction of product use, as in the cases of Lotronex, Cisapride, and Premarin.

Passive Surveillance

PMS falls into two categories—passive and active—depending upon the design of the activity. In passive PMS, physicians or patients initiate notification of an adverse event to an authority or the manufacturer. The spontaneous adverse event reporting systems offered by most regulatory agencies, such as MedWatch and ADRAC, are examples of passive PMS. Some companies provide prescribers with notification hotlines in the event that particular adverse events occur in association with their products. Unfortunately, passive PMS leads to significant underreporting of adverse events and often results in the collection of large amounts of dubious quality data that cannot be easily verified or followed up. Because passive surveillance does not track patient exposure, it is difficult to use this approach to establish the incidence of a particular side effect.

Active Surveillance

Active PMS, on the other hand, refers to a process in which adverse events are actively identified as part of a structured research activity. Active PMS is much better than the passive approach at accurately capturing representative safety data, but it requires a considerably greater investment of time, effort, and money from manufacturers and prescribers. Active PMS can be conducted as part of a post-marketing randomized clinical trial that evaluates, among other things, the safety of a product relative to placebo or other competitive treatments.

MONITORING PRODUCT SAFETY
Challenged by muscle-related safety concerns about Crestor, their new "statin," AstraZeneca invested in a series of pharma-coepidemiological studies to supplement data from their clinical trials and spontaneous adverse event reports. One of these studies was an active surveillance program conducted through the Drug Safety Research Unit in Southampton (UK) to monitor the safety of Crestor in the primary care setting. General practitioners were sent a green form for each of their patients approximately six months after their initiation with Crestor. The study, which collected data from an interim cohort of 2,722 patients revealed no cases of myopathy, myositis, or rhabdomyolysis.[1]

Although the studies that triggered Merck's Vioxx withdrawal and Premarin's demise were randomized clinical trials designed to investigate expanded efficacy benefits, they also represented examples of active PMS because they included safety outcomes data and adverse event collection. More often than not, however, active PMS is conducted as a special case of a product registry or an observational study with an explicit focus on drug safety. These are sometimes referred to as Post Marketing Surveillance Studies (PMSS) and Safety Surveillance Plans (SSP).

Investigator Dynamics

Most active PMS programs are conducted as special observational studies. They invite inclusion of patients who have started on the study drug within a certain period of time. PMS studies tend to have less restrictive inclusion/exclusion criteria than other studies, but they often need to capture patient disease, medical, and demographic characteristics to support appropriate analysis.

With some rare regional exceptions, observational PMS studies do not require sponsors to provide study drug, even though some studies involve scheduled visits as part of their design. Deviations from a naturalistic design can significantly impact the complexity of a study and the speed of the ethics/IRB approval process. PMS studies rarely offer patients any benefit (unless regular tests or reviews are included), and the focus of their design on long-term safety does not promise much immediate scientific immediacy. Successful implementation of a PMS study therefore requires extreme protocol simplicity and workflow sensitivity for data collection. Important also, are additional motivators, such as:

· · · · ·

Regulatory mandate. Countries such as Japan now mandate that physicians participate in PMS when prescribing recently approved products. Mandated PMS for new products can delay market adoption as prescribers avoid administrative workload by continuing to prescribe the older product rather than trying the new one.

Additional analyses. Supplementing the study with some additional observational data collection to increase scientific immediacy can significantly increase investigator participation. This is also a helpful approach for sponsors wishing to balance information about potential safety issues with information about potential benefits.

Investigator payment. It is often not possible for sponsors to improve the scientific immediacy or offer any significant benefit to patients for participation. Even when workload has been reduced to a minimum through simplified consent and batched follow-up processes, investigators often require greater-than-expected payment to ensure optimal site performance.

Pitfalls and Regulatory Issues

PMS studies are associated with simplified data collection, often to the exclusion of data that could be used to support non-safety related analyses. Because these studies offer little patient benefit and are of only limited immediate scientific interest, investigators often require significant payment for participation. This combination of high investigator payments, minimal workload, and linkage to the prescription of a particular product explains why, historically, PMS designs have been used to justify seeding studies.

Seeding studies have increasingly attracted negative attention, with many countries now imposing penalties against pharmaceutical companies performing this kind of activity. In the United

States, the Anti-kickback statute imposes significant financial and criminal penalties on companies and individuals involved in this type of activity (see appendix).

Unfortunately, by their very design, legitimate safety surveillance studies can be difficult to differentiate from nefarious ones. To make clear that a PMS study is not a seeding study, designers must pay particular attention to detail. They must document the safety purpose of the study. (Receiving a regulatory request to conduct such a study certainly helps!) Wherever possible, conduct a feasibility study across 10 to 20 sites to establish a fair and documented market rate for investigator payment. In addition, appropriately communicating results helps to establish the scientific credibility of the program.

References

1. Kasliwal RK, Wilton L, Shakir SAW. Safety profile of rosuvastatin as used in general practice in England: Interim results of a prescription-event monitoring study. Drug Safety 2004;27 (12): 939.

15   Conclusion: In the Wake of Vioxx

THE PUBLIC DEBATE SURROUNDING Merck's withdrawal of Vioxx in the fall of 2004 has been a wake-up call for regulatory authorities and the pharmaceutical industry, both of which had largely attempted to continue with business as usual after a string of high profile withdrawals that included Fen-Phen, Baycol, and Cisapride. Although I have already touched briefly on the Vioxx episode earlier in the book, I have reserved a fuller discussion of its implications for the industry for this more speculative concluding chapter—recognizing that an assessment of Vioxx and the entire COX2 market is far from over as I write this in May 2005.

Background

In the fall of 2004, Dr. David Graham's attention-grabbing retrospective investigation of Vioxx safety brought national publicity and focused intense scrutiny on selective COX2 inhibitors, a new generation of non-steroidal anti-inflammatory drugs (NSAIDs) associated with fewer gastrointestinal side effects than older agents.[1] Older NSAIDs—aspirin, naproxen, and ibuprofen—had revolutionized the treatment of pain and inflammation, bringing relief to patients with colds, headaches, and muscle pains, as well as to those suffering from more debilitating conditions such as osteoarthritis, rheumatoid arthritis and cancer. Unfortunately, these older painkillers had an unwanted action on the COX1 enzymes responsible for protecting the gastrointestinal tract—exposing hundreds of thousands of patients to a variety of side effects, ranging from dyspepsia to ulcer perforation and death. In 1997 more than 16,500 Americans died as a result of NSAID-induced gastrointestinal complications.[2]

The launch of Vioxx and Celebrex in 1999 seemed another leap forward in the management of pain and inflammation. These new painkillers selectively inhibited the COX2 enzyme responsible for inflammation without significantly inhibiting the gastro-protective COX1 enzyme. Based on claims of improved tolerability and safety, doctors began prescribing Vioxx and Celebrex in record numbers, with Vioxx generating almost $1 billion dollars in U.S. sales for Merck within its first year on the market.

By early 2000, however, the first questions began to appear about the cardiovascular safety of COX2 inhibitors. Preliminary data from the Phase IIIB VIGOR (Vioxx Gastrointestinal Outcomes Research) trial, a Merck-sponsored RCT comparing treatment with high-dose 50mg Vioxx against 500mg naproxen, identified a strong potential cardiovascular safety signal by demonstrating that patients receiving Vioxx were at four to five times the risk of having a heart attack versus those receiving the naproxen.[3]

Merck immediately went into damage control, defending the cardiovascular safety profile of Vioxx by suggesting that the VIGOR results demonstrated a cardioprotective effect of naproxen rather than an increased risk for Vioxx. At the same time, Merck began a number of new research activities which included a long-term Phase IIIB randomized, double-blind, placebo-controlled trial known as APPROVe which investigated a new indication for Vioxx as well as tracked data on cardiovascular safety concerns.

In the absence of any conclusive evidence to support its explanation of the VIGOR data, Merck began to face mounting pressure from regulators to reevaluate its product. In December 2000, the

FDA wrote to Merck expressing its concern about how the company was promoting the VIGOR results to the medical community. Members of the FDA Arthritis Advisory Committee extensively discussed the safety implications of the VIGOR study in February 2001 and reached an agreement with Merck to negotiate changes to the Vioxx label reflecting the cardiovascular uncertainty presented by the VIGOR data. In September 2001, the FDA wrote a warning letter to Merck highlighting concern that the company was claiming unsubstantiated superiority for Vioxx as well as minimizing cardiovascular safety results by omitting important risk information in their marketing activities.[4] After almost a year of negotiation over the wording, in April 2002 Merck added cardiovascular safety information to the Vioxx product label. The COX2 market continued to grow, and public discussion regarding Vioxx safety went quiet.

But in August 2004, FDA scientist Dr. David Graham dashed any hopes that the cardiovascular concerns over Vioxx were diminishing when he presented data from his retrospective case-control analysis of Kaiser Permanente patient records at the International Conference on Pharmacoepidemiology.[5] Dr. Graham's study, a Phase IV retrospective case-control analysis of Kaiser Permanente patient records, reidentified the safety signal associated with high-dose Vioxx use that had been originally detected four years earlier in the VIGOR trial. The study also suggested that a significant difference in cardiovascular risk could exist between Vioxx and its competitor, Celebrex. Graham's presentation triggered a frenzy of media activity and public concern.

Merck maintained its position that the VIGOR data did not indicate increased cardiovascular risk of Vioxx treatment until the week before the drug's withdrawal from the market in September 2004—when its APPROVe study's External Data Safety Monitoring Board notified the company of its recommendation to stop the study on the basis of cardiovascular safety. Facing another strong safety signal from within its own Phase IIIB randomized, double-blind, placebo-controlled data, Merck acted quickly to withdraw Vioxx worldwide in less than a week, overseeing the biggest pharmaceutical product recall in history.

Implications for the Pharmaceutical Industry

Over the past year, in light of Dr. Graham's Kaiser analysis, the Vioxx withdrawal, and considerable scientific and public discussion, I have faced two recurring questions from regulators, politicians, lawyers, and sponsors, both of which I feel are appropriate to reflect upon in concluding a handbook on strategic research in 2005.

1. Can Phase IV retrospective analysis of claims databases represent a quicker and cheaper alternative to prospective studies for monitoring drug safety?

2. What safety measures will drug companies and regulators be taking to protect patients and minimize medicolegal risk in the post-Vioxx climate?

Using administrative databases for safety surveillance

Having been involved in many retrospective epidemiological studies over the past five years, I have been consistently disappointed by both the appropriateness and completeness of administrative data available for retrospective safety-related data analysis. Although these datasets are a byproduct of the health insurance process, promising large amounts of data at very low cost, it is my experience that their current potential for safety signal sensitivity and specificity compares unfavorably with spontaneous adverse event reporting databases and cumulative meta-analysis of prospective observational and randomized controlled studies. The use of these administrative databases for safety signal detection and validation is in its infancy, and while improvements in the depth of data available and methodologies for analysis continue to be made, their existing limitations support their use as an adjunct tool for informing safety-decision making rather than as a primary screening system for safety surveillance.

The largest and most complete administrative databases available today are usually medical claims-related datasets that contain reliable information about patient age, sex, race, medication history, hospitalizations, medical procedures, and death but unfortunately very little else. They do not consistently include diagnoses, laboratory test results, and markers of disease activity, and when they do there is often pressure on healthcare providers to over-report diagnosis codes to maximize claim benefits.

When appropriate data is not available, epidemiologists are forced to use indirect methods to get the information they need. For example, they may use the prescription of an insulin or sulphonylurea as an indicator of diabetes, or the prescription of antibiotics as an indicator of infection. Because these indirect methods are not sensitive, investigators may miss many early signals (e.g., type II diabetes, diagnosed and managed by a family practitioner through diet and exercise, may never be recorded in a claims database). Because these markers are not specific (e.g., there are many reasons why a patient may commence ACE inhibitor treatment), it can be difficult for researchers to isolate meaningful signals amidst a sea of statistical background noise. In addition, it is my experience that these databases can experience attrition of 10 to 20 percent of their patients annually, with many patients lost to follow-up without any explanation for their disappearance. U.S.-based databases appear to have the largest attrition rates as patients move in and out of insurance networks when their employment circumstances change.

Analysts compensate for the combination of low sensitivity, low specificity, and suboptimal data completeness by requiring enormous volumes of data. Dr. Graham's retrospective analysis of 1,394,764 Kaiser Permanente patient health records, designed to confirm (rather than discover) the presence of a safety signal, still required three years worth of data from one of the largest and most complete data sets in the country, for one of the most prescribed drugs on the market, to simply establish what the Phase IV randomized controlled VIGOR trial had demonstrated four years earlier—that high-dose Vioxx treatment may be associated with an increased risk of cardiovascular disease. In addition, Dr. Graham's approach required data from at least another year of market experience to replicate the safety signal observed earlier in VIGOR. Even so, since only a small number of patients in the Kaiser database had experienced a heart attack and received high dose Vioxx treatment, the study was not able to define this increased risk within a tight confidence interval. Despite the attention the popular press devoted to the Graham study, most industry analysts agree that the strength of its conclusions alone may not have justified the withdrawal of Vioxx—and certainly not at standard doses.

In contrast to Dr. Graham's claims database approach, Peter Jüni and colleagues from the universities of Berne and Bristol conducted a cumulative meta-analysis of data from published prospective randomized and observational trials. Their findings, published by *Lancet* in December 2004, showed that an increased risk of heart attacks should have become evident by the end of 2000.[6] This meta-analysis showed that by the time 20,742 patients had been randomized to studies, and 52 heart attacks had occurred in these patients, it was possible to detect the increased relative cardiovascular risk for patients receiving Vioxx with much greater confidence, and with much lower margin for error than Dr. Graham's study. Somewhat shockingly, the meta-analysis found no evidence to suggest that Vioxx's cardiovascular toxicity was limited to long-term use or was dose dependent. The Jüni study attests to the possibility of conclusiveness in prospective research, particularly when a number of studies can be analyzed together.

Reviewing Dr. Graham's retrospective analysis in the context of Dr. Jüni's findings highlights the limitations of administrative data sets for safety analysis in their current form. If an analysis of data one of the largest and most complete administrative databases in the United States, relating to three years of prescribing history for a blockbuster product, could not identify a safety signal with the same clarity and conclusiveness as a meta-analysis of prospective studies that could have been done less than two years post launch, it is unrealistic—in my opinion—to expect that automated retrospective analysis of any administrative data set can be a viable alternative to prospective research for active safety surveillance at this time.

Proactive Safety Measures in the Post-Vioxx Environment

Although courts will be left to decide whether Merck applied the best practices of the time in their handling of Vioxx safety, the level of public discussion surrounding the Vioxx withdrawal has definitively raised public expectations for best practice in drug-safety monitoring going forward. Even as agencies and politicians debate possible changes in the regulatory environment, medicolegal fears are already changing industry practices in a way that additional regulation can only serve to reinforce. Both forces are driving demand for more Phase IIIB and IV prospective research to study safety and more Phase IV risk management programs to increase protection for patients.

Regulators are facing the impossible task of responding to drug safety challenges brought to a head by the Vioxx withdrawal while attempting to reignite industry innovation. Since 2000, the number of investigational new drug applications and new drug approvals has declined, mainly because of the increasing costs of developing drugs and the increasing chance that research programs will fail to produce a marketable drug. With the average cost of carrying a successful compound through Phases I–III doubling over the past five years, most regulators are loathe to add greater complexity, duration, and cost to the drug development process. Instead they are focusing on ways to allow earlier approval, if appropriate risk management procedures are in place.

1. Increased Focus on Post-marketing Prospective Research

Regulators are already demanding that sponsors commit to research on important potential risks and investigate important missing information as a condition of approval. In the United States, more than 73 percent of new drug approvals are associated with one or more Phase IV research commitments.[7] In Europe, the EMEA negotiates detailed pharmacovigilance plans with sponsors before approval, which describe the routine safety monitoring activities to be offered by the sponsor as well as studies and milestones that a sponsor commits to as a condition of approval.

Whereas spontaneous adverse event collection and retrospective monitoring of administrative databases will continue to serve as valuable tools in support of safety decision-making, prospective research—either conducted as Phase IIIB and IV randomized controlled trials or observational studies designed to capture data from a broader patient population—represents the gold standard for informing safety decision-making. In the current environment, manufacturers are already finding it hard to justify the medicolegal risk of relying on less sensitive and specific methodologies in Phase IIIB and IV as a substitute for additional prospective research. In addition, many companies are taking a fresh look at their commitment study plans on the basis that delays could suggest less than best efforts in pharmacovigilance even in the absence of regulatory powers to enforce the timely completion of Phase IV studies.

In the past, Phase IIIB and IV studies conducted by the same sponsor varied significantly in the standards they applied to the collection of safety data, making it more difficult to perform the type of cumulative meta-analysis conducted by Jüni for Vioxx. The bulk of this research work was conducted through small CROs and academic research groups with differing (and sometimes non-existent) standards for data management, adverse event documentation and monitoring. This made it almost impossible for sponsors to maintain consistency. A number of companies have already chosen to outsource adverse event processing for their post-marketing studies on a functional rather than project-by-project basis to ensure standardization. Others are attempting to achieve the same effect by reducing the number of Phase IIIB and IV service providers they use while focusing their internal efforts on ongoing analyses of accumulating safety data to avoid being beaten to a conclusion by an outside party.

2. Appropriate Use / Patient Risk Management Programs

Patient risk management programs are designed primarily for the protection of individual patients. Although data is usually pooled for safety analysis, like in the Phase IV safety studies discussed in the previous section, this is usually a secondary objective of most risk management programs.

Other industries, such as the baby products and car manufacturing industries, already have consumer risk management programs in place: manufacturers of baby products are required to provide consumer registration services in order to track buyers in the event of a product recall; and car manufacturers not only track the buyers of their vehicles, but also subsidize early warranty services to ensure that their cars are working safely and that necessary repairs are conducted early in case a fault is found.

A number of large pharmaceutical companies are already beginning to consider structured risk management programs for patients receiving their products. Companies are starting to offer patients access to programs that are a combination of a patient tracking service, health education initiative, patient risk management program and an active Phase IV safety surveillance study. Patients enrolling in these programs gain access to regular communications about their disease, new efficacy and safety information about their drug (including changes in the recommended use of a product), and subsidized investigations such as liver function tests, X-Rays, and antibody tests.

For example, a manufacturer of a new product that has not yet established its cardiovascular safety in a large population may choose to offer patients access to yearly stress electrocardiogram testing, a simple screening test that insurance companies would be hesitant to cover in these circumstances. Or by maintaining a patient list, a pharmaceutical manufacturer would be able to conduct a selective product recall by notifying affected patients and their doctors on an individual basis in the event that new information surfaces suggesting an unfavorable risk / benefit profile for a particular patient subpopulation.

Sponsors that conduct these programs can also ensure that their products are being largely used as recommended, and—by monitoring the level and significance of off-label prescribing—can take action if further Phase IIIB research, regulatory filing, or medical communications are necessary to ensure that doctors are well informed of the risks associated with a particular pattern of off-label prescribing. In addition, they can also prospectively collect patient safety and outcomes data for ongoing, high quality safety analysis.

By monitoring appropriate use, testing patients for potential side-effects, and collecting large amounts of safety-focused prospective data, sponsors can quickly and cheaply demonstrate a commitment to patient safety that meets the standards already set by other industries. Perhaps Vioxx would still be on the market—albeit restricted to a narrower patient population—had Merck put a risk management program in place in 2000. It would have allowed them to (1) identify patients at low risk for gastrointestinal side-effects and high risk for cardiovascular disease that could be inappropriately receiving Vioxx in light of the VIGOR data and (2) offer regular subsidized cardiac stress testing or other screening services to patients that continued with Vioxx treatment.

3. Probationary Approval

No product approved by the FDA in the last 10 years has involved more than 25,000 patients in registration studies. To do so would delay approval of most drugs by 2 to 5 years and add over $100 million to the cost of drug development. In the case of specialty medications for diseases with relatively targeted patient populations, such as certain cancers and autoimmune diseases, establishing safety in large populations could delay approval by decades. Such delays would degrade patients' access to treatment, and—by delaying sales opportunities for pharmaceutical manufacturers—reduce industry enthusiasm for drug development.

Recognizing how aggressively Vioxx and other COX2 inhibitors were promoted (and adopted) post-launch, despite a limited understanding of their safety profile, regulators now feel pressure to rein in pharmaceutical marketing activities until a product's safety profile is better characterized. Some industry analysts are predicting that regulators could opt for a probationary stage of drug approval as a compromise between the demand for more pre-approval safety data and concern over increased drug development costs and delays. A probationary approval stage could reduce the time to market for new products by making them available under tightly controlled conditions as soon as their Phase III research program comes to a close. During this period, prescribing would be limited to patients that meet strict inclusion/exclusion criteria (e.g., no "off-label" prescribing). Manufacturers could profit from product sales but would be unable to conduct direct-to-consumer marketing, or any form of product promotion or detailing. Finally, regulators would require that manufacturers provide the probationary product through a patient risk management program that included reporting safety data back to the regulatory agency on a frequent basis.

Creating a probationary approval stage would allow regulators to demand much larger amounts of Phase IIIB safety data as a condition of marketing authorization without compromising patient access to new treatments or stifling the industry's ability to generate revenue. Proponents of a probationary approval stage argue that this approach would protect patient safety by ensuring that early access to new medications would take place under tightly controlled safety conditions. In addition it would encourage the movement of new products through the development pipeline by shortening the period between drug discovery and sales by one to two years.

Conclusion

In response to a safety analysis performed on their own research study, Merck voluntarily announced their decision to withdraw Vioxx from the market on September 30, 2004. The event led to an immediate 26 percent drop in Merck's stock and the beginning of front-page media attention focused on the entire COX2 market.

The broader impact of Vioxx's withdrawal will not be known for years to come, but it is clear that we are already starting to see the direction of long-term changes in the pharmaceutical industry as attention is focused on prospective Phase IIIB and IV research, Phase IV risk management programs, and ways to promote earlier access to new treatments while increasing patient safety. Those working in the field of Phase IIIB and IV research need to be prepared for these changes and remain abreast of developments as they emerge.

References

1. Memorandum from David J. Graham to Paul Seligman, MD, MPH, Acting Director, Office of Drug Safety, Risk of acute myocardial infarction and sudden cardiac death in patients treated with COX-2 selective and non-selective NSAIDs. 30 September 2004, available at http://www.fda.gov/cder/drug/infopage/vioxx/vioxxgraham.pdf.*

2. Singh G, Triadafilopoulos, G. Epidemiology of NSAID-induced gastrointestinal complications. J Rheumatol 1999;26(Suppl 56):18-24.

3. Bombardier C, et al., Comparison of upper gastrointestinal toxicity of rofecoxib and naproxen in patients with rheumatoid arthritis. VIGOR Study Group, N Engl J Med 2000 Nov 23;343(21):1520-8.

4. Warning Letter to Mr. Raymond Gilmartin, Department of Human Services, September 2001, available at http://www.fda.gov/foi/warning_letters/g1751d.htm.*

5. Memorandum from David J. Graham to Paul Seligman, MD, MPH, Acting Director, Office of Drug Safety, Risk of Acute Myocardial Infarction and Sudden Cardiac Death in Patients Treated with COX-2 Selective and Non-Selective NSAIDs, 30 September 2004, available at http://www.fda.gov/cder/drug/infopage/vioxx/vioxxgraham.pdf.*

6. Jüni P, et al., Risk of cardiovascular events and rofecoxib: cumulative meta-analysis. Lancet 2004 December 4;364(2021-29).

7. Tufts CSDD Impact Report. FDA request post-marketing studies in 73% of recent drug approvals. July-August 2004. 6(4), available at http://csdd.tufts.edu/InfoServices/ImpactReportPDFs/ ImpRptJulyAug2005.pdf.*

*Note: All citations to websites listed in this book were verified in May of 2005.

APPENDIX
Anti-Kickback
Statute and False
Claims Act*

Note: This appendix applies to research activities conducted within the United States. Regulations relating to the promotion of pharmaceutical products, and any associated conduct of clinical research, differ between countries and regions.

Background

The Office of the Inspector General (OIG) at Health and Human Services (HHS) in Washington, D.C., oversees compliance with the Anti-kickback statute (AKS) and the False Claims Act (FCA). In May 2003, the office released guidance on these statutes and on continuing medical education. This guidance, along with the Department of Justice's increased prosecution of alleged violations under these laws, indicates that the government is vigorously prosecuting under these statutes and widening their application. The OIG has also made clear that, in its view, a violation of the Anti-kickback statute may also give rise to False Claim Act liability under certain circumstances.

* I thank Nancy Strehlow and Judith Beach for providing the information for this chapter. Much of the content is based on their presentation on the Anti-kickback statute to the DIA in June of 2004.

Section 1128(b) of the Social Security Act, (the Anti-kickback statute or AKS), provides for criminal penalties for certain acts impacting Medicare and other reimbursable services. This statute makes it a felony for any person to "knowingly and willfully" offer to pay another person as an inducement for referring patients to products or services that will be paid for by a government health-care program. Penalties include fines in the millions of dollars, exclusion from federal programs, and jail time.

The False Claims Act (FCA) prohibits the "knowing" submission of false claims to obtain payment from the government. The FCA includes significant mandatory civil penalties of at least $10,000 per violation (in the case of clinical research this is per falsely claimed prescription) plus three times damage. The FCA allows an individual acting as a "whistleblower," who knows about any person or entity who is submitting false claims, to bring a suit on behalf of the government and share in any damages recovered as a result.

Recent lawsuits under these statutes have resulted in settlements of $875 million by TAP Pharmaceuticals in 2001, $622 million by Abbott Laboratories in 2003, and $430 million by Pfizer in 2004.

The Anti-Kickback Statute and Strategic Research

Any study that involves both the payment of a physician and the prescription of a government-funded pharmaceutical product has the potential to be misconstrued as a framework for paying physicians to write prescriptions. This risk applies even when the manufacturer provides a pharmaceutical product free of charge for the period of the study, if ongoing use would still be required once the study is over. Because these conditions apply for almost all Phase

IIIB and IV studies, understanding of the AKS and its application to clinical research is critical for anyone planning to conduct strategic research in the United States.

Of central importance to the statute is the concept of "knowingly" attempting to "induce" physicians to prescribe a government-reimbursed product, resulting in the following key implications:

- Just because a study gathers data supporting a product's competitive position does not automatically implicate it as an inducement to prescribe.

- Just because a study has a valid scientific objective does not automatically exclude the possibility of inducement being a parallel objective (one-purpose rule).

- Phase IIIB and IV research, which involves products that are either reimbursed or expect reimbursement in the near-term from government agencies, is at greater risk of AKS exposure than registration research.

Whether or not there are legitimate scientific reasons for the study, if one of the purposes of the study is to induce purchase of the drug, you can be prosecuted under AKS. Any party associated with the study whom the OIG can demonstrate was "knowingly" involved in the inducement to prescribe can be held liable under the AKS.

As an example, if a sponsor pays investigators $500 per patient "enrolled" in a simple data collection study with the intent that this payment be used as an incentive for doctors to enroll 20,000 patients on study medication, the court can find the sponsor guilty under the statute, and require them to pay $500 million in fines ($25,000 per violation times 20,000 violations). Jail time for executives and exclusion from Medicare (the "death sentence") is also possible. For obvious reasons, the AKS has virtually eliminated the once common industry practice of conducting "seeding studies" in the U.S. market. The fact that this practice was once considered routine in the industry does not exempt it from prosecution.

High Risk Activities

Studies that require switching products on initiation
Single arm, observational studies that require switching from one medication to another are at very high risk under the AKS—particularly if they involve large investigator payments.

Studies that involve large investigator payments
Payments to investigators must be limited to reasonable compensation for services provided. Any amount above this is presumed to be for the purpose of inducing the sales of the drug.

Studies with excessively large sample sizes
Sample sizes must be limited to statistically justifiable numbers for any post-registration research study. Any amount above this can be presumed to be for the purpose of inducing sales. Large samples are frequently used to allow for sub-analysis of different population groups. If this is the case, ensure it is documented as part of the statistical analysis plan before commencing the study.

Studies with questionable scientific value
Studies of questionable scientific value were identified by the OIG in a "Special Fraud Alert" as studies that warrant prosecution. Even if studies have a clear scientific purpose, you can still be prosecuted if one of the purposes of the study is to induce sales of the drug.

Studies directed by marketing
Recent federal guidance on this issue states, "Studies that originate or are directed by sales or marketing groups—are considered

particularly suspect …. Prudent manufacturers will develop contracting procedures that clearly separate the awarding of research contracts from marketing" (CPG, 20-21).[1]

Safe Harbours

Safe harbors are HHS regulations that identify practices that do not violate the AKS. You are protected from prosecution if you meet these additional requirements for safe harbors. As of the writing of this book, there is no safe harbor for participating in clinical research; as a result most people recommend ensuring that post-marketing research activities are designed to come as close as possible to complying with the "personal services and management" safe harbor.

Checklist for Compliance within AKS and the Personal Services and Management Safe Harbor

- *Are you keeping payments consistent?* Payments must be consistent among similarly situated investigators. High prescribers must not be rewarded by higher payments.

- *Are you providing compensation only?* No gifts or honorariums. No payment should be provided for any purpose other than services.

- *Have you stated a clear scientific purpose?* The sponsor must clearly identify the purpose of the study, the sponsor's scientists must review and analyze the results, and the researchers must send out the study for consideration for publication.

- *Do you have a written protocol that specifies investigator duties and protects patients?* The protocol must identify investigator's services and show that these are necessary to accomplish study goals. Have HIPAA authorizations and/or informed consents in place if necessary. Obtain IRB review by a central, independent IRB or a commercial IRB.

- *Are you paying reasonable compensation?* Payments must be fair market value (FMV), and you must document the calculation of FMV.

- *Are you conducting the study separate from any marketing activities?* The study must be conducted by researchers not marketing personnel.

- *Are you selecting investigators based on research needs?* Investigators must be selected on rational, documented criteria that support the purpose of the study. Researchers rather than marketing personnel must select investigators.

- *Have you established a reasonable study size?* Verify that the number of patients and sites is required by the study and document this process.

- *Have you signed specific, written agreements with all investigators?* The site contract should list investigator duties, require the investigator to follow the protocol, state that the investigator's judgment is not affected by the compensation, and specify the amount of compensation.

- *Have you set a one-year investigator agreement term?* A full one-year term is required by the Personal Service Safe Harbor, but post-marketing studies often do not last a year. Include a clause that the term is the "longer of" one year or time to complete the study.

- *Have you ensured that the investigator agreement covers all services?*

- *Have you set the payments for each site service?* Verify that the total payments for each service, per patient, are the same for all sites. Verify that these payments were set in advance, and, if possible, pay at pre-determined intervals.

- *Have you verified that you are not setting different payments for higher subscribers?* No bonuses are allowed for higher volume sites.

- *Have you verified that you are not promoting or condoning illegal activities?* These include violations under the FCA and off-label promotion regulations.

False Claims Act and Strategic Research

It is illegal to knowingly make false claims to the government for the reimbursement of drugs or to use a false record to get a false claim paid. Although CROs and pharmaceutical companies do not make claims directly to the government for drugs, the OIG argues that clinical trials that constitute a violation of the AKS also constitute a violation of the FCA.

Half of the courts have accepted this OIG argument; the other half believes the liability resides with the health care providers themselves. Be that as it may, to date courts have awarded hundreds of millions of dollars to the government for violation of the FCA in post-marketing studies.

Under the FCA the person who turns in the company gets up to 15 to 20 percent of settlement. Whistleblowers have reaped tens of millions of dollars for turning companies in. One vice-president of sales wore a wiretap for years, was rewarded with millions by the federal government, and then went and collected an additional $47.5 million for being a whistleblower at his next employer. While these rich rewards would probably not stand up in appeals to the top courts, no company has been brave enough to present the legal challenge.

High Risk Activities

Off-Label Promotion Regulations

Phase IIIB studies in which an approved product is being investigated for unapproved indication may be perceived as promoting off-label use of the product. When performing these studies ensure that investigators are selected on the basis of their ability to conduct the research and not on their prescribing activity. Ensure that the intent to investigate a possible label change is well documented, and that procedures implemented to monitor Phase IIIB protocols also include oversight of investigator trial activities.

Billing for free product

Site agreements or contracts should clearly remind sites that it is illegal to bill Medicare/Medicaid or other third parties for products that the CRO or sponsor provides as part of the study. As part of the on-site monitoring process, it is prudent for CRAs to ensure that sites are operating in compliance with this directive.

Billing for study-specific services

Site agreements or contracts should clearly remind sites that it is illegal to bill Medicare/Medicaid or other third parties for services for which the CRO or sponsor will reimburse as part of the study. Ask the question, "Would I perform the procedure if the study was not going on?" The protocol and budget must be specific about what are study-specific services because it is often common for a consultation to include both a study related component as well as other clinical care activities. For example, a patient attending a physician for treatment of a sore throat may be enrolled in a clinical trial for a new antiseptic gargle. The physician is reimbursed for identifying, consenting, and initiating the patient on the study, but the initial consultation resulting in the diagnosis of acute pharyngitis is usually not paid for by a study sponsor.

Lack of informed consent

Studies funded in part by government grants may give rise to FCA violations if appropriate informed consent is not sought from patients. One U.S. Attorney has publicly suggested that since the government would not fund studies that lack informed consent, any study that obtained funding without appropriate informed consent could constitute a false claim. No cases have been brought yet under this interpretation, however, in February of 2005, a large university paid in excess of $500,000 to settle a claim by the federal government that alleged inadequacies in the university's informed consent and screening processes in a study funded by the National Institute of Health violated the False Claims Act.

Checklist For False Claims Act

- *Do you adequately train all staff regarding off-label promotion rules?* Document training and keep it up-to-date, since CRAs frequently have little exposure to promotional rules and regulations.

- *Do you include a "no billing for free products" provision in investigator agreements?* Good practice involves including provisions in site contracts and in the site/investigator training program.

- *Do you ensure that reimbursement advice is appropriate?*

- *Have you avoided any AKS violations?* Ensure compliance with the AKS (see section above) to avoid triggers for the False Claims Act.

- *Have you verified that your informed consents are sufficient?*

If your staff reports a violation of either of these statutes, you must never retaliate against the person who brought it to your attention.

Do not refuse to cooperate with the government because this can look like concealment. Do not try to influence a whistleblower because you can be charged with fraud or concealment.

Summary

When outsourcing strategic research, ensure the CROs you select (1) specialize in Phase IIIb and IV research, (2) have specialized SOPs designed to ensure compliance with the Anti-kickback statute and the False Claims Act, and (3) have adequate training and quality assurance measures in place to support their SOPs. Since penalties for violations can seriously damage a company financially, it is essential that sponsors regularly audit their providers to ensure that these three standards are met. Sponsors can be held liable for violations of these statutes even if they do not perform the clinical study themselves. Do not think that giving the study to someone else to perform gets you off the hook.

References

1. Office of Inspector General's Compliance Program Guidance for Pharmaceutical Manufacterers. *Federal Register*, Vol. 68, No. 86, page 23731, Monday, May 5, 2003.

Glossary

active surveillance. The process of obtaining follow-up safety information from patients that have received treatment through methods that include observational studies, randomized trials, or frequent automated monitoring of administrative claims databases.

Anti-kickback statute (AKS). Applied to the pharmaceutical industry, the US statute (42 USC §1320a-7b) treats as a crime any inducement to physicians to prescribe drugs or other medical products that will be reimbursed by government insurance plans. Phase IIIB and IV clinical trials can fall afoul of this legislation if one of the purposes of any payment to investigators is to get them to prescribe the study product and the study product may be reimbursed by the government.

approved medical products. Those that have received marketing authorization.

brand team. A group of representatives from different pharmaceutical functions (such as medical affairs, marketing and sales) who collectively set priorities and strategies for a particular medical product, including directions for potential research.

case report form (CRF). A paper or electronic document upon which investigators can record patient data relating to a clinical trial.

clinical study. Any research activity that investigates the use of medical products that do not involve the trial of a treatment, including activities such as registries or retrospective studies. See *clinical trial.*

clinical trial. A program evaluating the effectiveness, safety, or action upon the human body of a medical treatment by testing its use in a group of patients which usually range in number from a few to thousands.

cohort. A group of study participants managed and followed in a similar way over the course of a study.

controlled trial. A clinical trial that allows the effectiveness and/or safety of one treatment to be compared against another (including placebo). Controlled trials attempt to keep constant potentially confounding characteristics between different treatment groups so that differences in patient outcomes can be attributed to differences in treatments received.

clinical research associate (CRA). A person that oversees the progress and conduct of clinical trials to ensure the speed and quality of data collected and protection of study subjects.

contract research organization (CRO). A business that provides clinical research related services to the pharmaceutical industry, e.g., running clinical trials, performing assays, identifying investigators, etc.

cross-sectional study. A study in which data is collected from subjects at a single point in time.

double-blind trial. A study in which neither the investigator or patient knows which treatment they are receiving.

electronic data capture (EDC). The collection of study data using personal computers, websites, or personal digital assistants (PDAs) rather than paper.

endpoints. The primary efficacy or safety characteristics of a treatment being assessed in a clinical study (such as mortality rate, number of hospitalizations, length of survival, cost of healthcare).

ethics committee (EC). See institutional review board (IRB).

European Clinical Trials Directive (EU-CTD). The European Union directive harmonizing the administrative provisions governing clinical trials across European countries.

European Agency for the Evaluation of Medicinal Products (EMEA). The regulatory agency that oversees medical product development and approval in the European Union.

European Union Privacy Directive. The European Union directive protecting the right to privacy with respect to the processing of personal data. This directive applies widely to all businesses, including clinical research.

expanded access programs. Programs that make promising, but unapproved, medical products available to patients with serious and life threatening illnesses. Also called early access or compassionate use programs.

False Claims Act (FCA). The act used to prosecute those who make false claims to the government for the reimbursement of medical treatments.

Food and Drug Administration (FDA). The US agency overseeing the regulation of drugs, medical products, cosmetics and foods.

Health and Human Service (HHS). The US agency that oversees Medicare and Medicaid. The HHS Office of Inspector General prosecutes cases involving application of the Anti-kickback statute and False Claims Act to the pharmaceutical industry

Health Insurance Portability and Accountability Act of 1996 (HIPAA). The US legislation that protects patients' privacy and ensures health insurance coverage when their circumstances change.

International Conference on Harmonization: Good Clinical Practice (ICH-GCP). The international ethical and scientific quality standard for the conduct of clinical trials involving human subjects agreed to by the International Conference on Harmonization in May 1996.

investigational new drug (IND) application. A request to conduct trials in human subjects involving a drug that is not approved, is being used for a non-approved indication, or is being administered in a non-approved formulation.

institutional review board (IRB). A committee that oversees clinical trials with the purpose of protecting the scientific quality and safety of subjects in a clinical trial. An IRB can approve, demand modifications to, or disapprove research.

marketing authorization. Permission granted by a regulatory agency to market and sell a medical product.

naturalistic study. A study that only requires standard medical management, investigations or physician visits. Also called an actual use or real world study because it does not interfere in any way with the real-world treatment and experience of the subject.

new drug application (NDA). The application submitted by a drug manufacturer requesting that the FDA consider a product for marketing authorization.

observational study. A study that observes the outcomes of treatment initiated through standard medical management (not as a result of randomization or other form of patient assignment). Unlike a naturalistic study, an observational study can involve a regular schedule for patient follow-up or the conduct of non-standard investigations (e.g., thrice-monthly cholesterol checks).

Office of the Inspector General (OIG). A team of attorneys within US government agencies responsible for prosecuting violations of federal laws that apply to their agency. The Health and Human

Services OIG prosecutes cases involving application of the Anti-kickback Statute and False Claims Act.

open-label study. A study in which both the investigator and subject know which product the subject is receiving.

passive surveillance. The process of obtaining safety information through spontaneous reporting of adverse events by physicians, patients and hospitals.

Phase I studies. The first trials of an investigational new drug in humans, they are conducted on patients or normal volunteer subjects and are designed to investigate toxicity, and how the drug is absorbed, distributed, and eliminated from the body.

Phase II studies. Well controlled, closely monitored studies that represent the first trials designed to establish efficacy of an investigational new drug in humans. Phase II trials are commonly used to establish an appropriate dose regime and short term side-effect profile in preparation for Phase III.

Phase III studies. Studies designed to establish the effectiveness and safety of an investigational new drug in humans. These are the final trials which support an application for marketing authorization.

Phase IIIB studies. Studies that occur after submission of an application for marketing authorization (but do not involve investigation of approved drugs for approved indications). Pre-approval Phase IIIB studies take place in the period between submission and approval of a new drug. Post-approval Phase IIIB studies investigate new indications once a product is already on the market.

Phase IV studies. Studies that investigate the use of approved products for approved indications. These studies include long-term safety studies (which can be required by regulatory agencies), studies to establish treatment guidelines, and studies that examine the use of the drug in different patient populations or at different stages of disease. Also known as post-marketing studies.

post-marketing safety studies (PMS). Ongoing studies designed to collect safety data relating to the use of a marketed product. Sometimes referred to as Post Marketing Surveillance Studies (PMSS) or Safety Surveillance Plans (SSP). See also active and passive surveillance.

post-marketing studies. See Phase IV studies

prospective study. A study in which subjects are enrolled and data collected going forward in time.

randomized controlled trial (RCT). A trial in which patients are assigned by chance to treatment groups, thereby maximizing the probability that patient groups are statistically similar in all ways except the treatment being investigated. In the book these are also referred to as experimental trials. See also controlled trial.

registration research. Clinical research conducted in support of an application for marketing authorization. This research occurs in Phase I, II, and III.

registry. A clinical study that passively collects data on patients suffering from a particular disease (disease registry), receiving a particular treatment (product registry) or connected by a common exposure (exposure registry). Often described as "looking over a doctor's shoulder", a registry is a prospective open-label observational study.

retrospective study. A study that involves analysis of previously captured data, such as a chart review of data recorded in patient files or an analysis of a pharmaceutical claims database.

single-blind study. A study in which only the investigator knows which treatment the patient is receiving *sponsor.* The organization that initiates and finances a clinical study.

standard operating procedure (SOP). For the purposes of this book, a written policy and procedure maintained by sponsors and CROs relating to the operational conduct of clinical trials.

statin (HMG-CoA reductase inhibitor). A type of drug that lowers cholesterol levels by inhibiting the HMG-CoA reductase enzyme involved in cholesterol synthesis.

strategic research. Clinical studies conducted to ensure that physicians, patients and payors have sufficient information to support optimal use of a marketed product. The term is used synonymously with Phase IIIB and IV trials which are performed after the submission of an application for marketing authorization.

unapproved medical products. Those that have not received marketing authorization.

Index

Glossary items listed in the index are indicated by **bold** typeface page references.

Photography and Design Credits

Cover photo: Nino Mascardi/Getty Images

Front cover concept: Jim Phillips

Cover and text design: Sarah Stengle

Interior Photos: pages 69 and 99, McIntyre Photography, Inc.